GW01397953

Jeanie Civil is a consultant psychologist, teacher, psychotherapist, BPS psychometric tester, broadcaster and author. She has considerable experience as a management trainer and her clients included medical, business, industrial and educational personnel. She worked for the National Further and Higher Education Management Staff College, Coombe Lodge, Lighthouse Professional Development for Teachers, Network Training SFE, CEM, Keystages and Style Women's Prison and numerous schools and FE and HE colleges. She was the CPD organiser and the Chair of Sussex Counselling and Psychotherapy.

She was the first woman ABBA coach and England Team Manager for Women's Basketball.

To Michael

with Thanks for cleaning my mind.

Much love

Civil

Jeanie

I dedicate this book to my son, Carl Damian Brookes, of whom I am so proud and love dearly.

I hope that this book brings him, and many others like him, who lost their parent when a child, acceptance, enlightenment, hope, laughter, happiness, inner peace and above all mental wellness.

Jeanie Civil

My Mind Made Me Me

How does your mind affect you?

AUSTIN MACAULEY PUBLISHERS™

LONDON * CAMBRIDGE * NEW YORK * SHARJAH

Copyright © Jeanie Civil 2023

The right of Jeanie Civil to be identified as author of this work has been asserted by the author in accordance with sections 77 and 78 of the Copyright, Designs and Patents Act 1988.

All rights reserved. No part of this publication may be reproduced, stored in a retrieval system, or transmitted in any form or by any means, electronic, mechanical, photocopying, recording, or otherwise, without the prior permission of the publishers.

Any person who commits any unauthorised act in relation to this publication may be liable to criminal prosecution and civil claims for damages.

A CIP catalogue record for this title is available from the British Library.

ISBN 9781035837083 (Paperback)
ISBN 9781035837090 (Hardback)
ISBN 9781035837106 (ePub e-book)

www.austinmacauley.com

First Published 2023
Austin Macauley Publishers Ltd®
1 Canada Square
Canary Wharf
London
E14 5AA

I would like to thank Austin Macauley Publishers, Carl Brookes, Brenda Mallon, Geoff Civil, Hugh Street, Judi Geisler, Jay Butler, Norman Dickie, Peter Wolfenden, Peter James, Richard Tuset, Simon Blacker and Dee Wood for their inspiration and their belief in me to be able and sufficiently qualified, to write this book. Thank you to Colum Clinton and Maria-Louise Maeder, for their digital prowess.

In addition, thank you to the thousands of students who questioned me, sought counselling and cried about their childhoods.

Also, my thanks go to the many anonymous clients who convinced me of just how important our childhoods are in affecting our thinking and our mental health, as they shared their secret anxieties and shame, in their search to find self-love.

Table of Contents

1. Introduction

Hello. Did your mind make you – you?

How was your mind influenced as a child?

Those early chilhood messages and experiences may stay with you for life but you can change them.

Were you born with a silver spoon in your mouth or, reflecting on your childhood, would you think that you had a rough ride of ridicule?

So many poems, posters and pamphlets have been designed to show us all how important our childhood experiences are in influencing our mind.

As a young nursery nurse I was so influenced by a Scottish Health Education poster, written anonymously, entitled 'If a child lives with ... he learns to ...', for instance that:

"If a child lives with *praise* he learns to *praise others*."

I recall now that the whole thing was about 'he', no mention of any 'she's' in the world.

I bravely said to our great very posh education tutor, "Why are they all 'he'?"

Her reply was, "All the books that we use, use 'he', so when you see 'he' – just think 'she'."

Researching now is mentally so much healthier, all genders can now relate to the message. He's and she's alternate in subsequent similar writings.

So I am adding and adapting to this idea of using the gist of this Scottish mental health poster warning of

"If as a child we lived:

With criticism, we learn to condemn;

with hostililily, we fight;

with ridicule, become shy;

with shame, become guilty;

with sexual abuse, become abusers;

with secrets, dishonest;

with bullying, a bully;

with divorce, fear of losing love;

with death, rejection;

with betrayal, lack of trust;

with anger, angry;

with violence, an agressor,

with racist comments, a racist;

with alchoholics, an alchoholic;

with drug abuse, an addict;

with mental illness, anxious.

Of course this is not inevitable, yes we really can all change our minds, feelings and behavour.

On the other hand if we lived as a child with positive messages and experiences, we would not want or need to change.

Hence, if as a child, we lived

with encouragement, we learn to be confident;

with tolerence, to be patient;

with praise, to be appreciative;

with approval, to feel self love;

with a loving religion, to be loving;

with honesty, to be truthful;

with friendliness, to believe that we are in a good place;

with acceptance, to feel valued;

with kindness, to be kind;

with genuiness, to trust

with calmness, to be mentally quiet;

with love, to love."

How far back can you remember? What 'scripts', messages, mantras or guidelines were you given as a small child ? As we move through this book, there may be sometimes when you will feel very happy, empathic, knowledgeable, sad, regretful perhaps, but you will always be given the opportunity to gain insight as to how you have come to feel, think and behave in the way that you do now, at whatever age you are presently. So let us begin by reflecting upon our childhood 'life scripts'.

2. Life Scripts

A life script is what is given to us in childhood, verbally or non-verbally, and may become a personal plan adopted by us, which often influences us and affects us in the way we think, feel, behave or the role we play with others.

Please start by filling in the following questionaire. Be honest, there is no point in being anything else, in order to gain personal insight into how your mind may have made you – you.

What did your parents, or significant adults in your life, say to you, verbally or nonverbally, about the following:

Your birth story? (You were a mistake, really wanted, how or where you were born, anything that you remember being told, named after you dead aunt who commited sucicide!)

How did they behave towards you when you were emotionally hurt?

How did they behave towards you when you were crying or upset?

How did they behave towards you when you were naughty?

If you had two significant adults in your early childhood did you feel loved by –

Both of them?   -----------------------------

One of them?   -----------------------------

Niether of them?   -----------------------------

What memories do have about how they treated your syblings, if applicable?

How does that make you feel now?

What were your first achievements?

What happened to you in your early childhood that made you feel different?

Did you ever feel special?

What made you happy as a child?

What did you want to do or be when you grew up?

Who did you want to be like?

Did any adult hurt or frighten you?

What did your parents or significant others say to you about;
Education?

Jealousy?

What kind of career you should train for or how you would 'end up'?

Politics?

Marriage?

Religion?

Sex?

Stealing?

Black people?

Assertiveness? (standing up for yourself)

Handling criticism?

Intelligence?

Money?

Bullying?

Death?

Love?

Now start by becoming aware of how you were affected by some of the things that you were told or you witnessed or you experienced as a child. Those family secrets that were told to you, or stories that you overheard. Looking at the content list, what do you think, feel or how do you already know how you think, feel or behave in some of those areas?

Which of the issues that we will be addressing in this book do you already think that you are skilled or knowledgeable about?

Make any notes of memories good or bad as you read through the chapters before we open up the gateways to your insight.

3. Your Memory Is in Your Brain

Although it may seem obvious, memory is formed within your brain. So anything that generally improves your brain health may also have a positive impact on your memory. Physical exercise and engaging in novel brain-stimulating activities – such as a crossword puzzle, bridge, chess or Sudoku – are a few proven methods for helping to keep your brain healthy.

There are two kinds of memory – short-term and long-term. Short-term memory is the kind of memory our brain uses to store small pieces of information needed right away, like someone's name or telephone number. Whereas long-term memory is for things you don't need to remember this instant, like all the memorable moments in your life. When you meet someone for the first time concentrate on them and on their name, not on yourself.

Stop wondering, *what are they thinking about me? My hair is a mess, I have egg on my shirt!*

New Academic Theories (NLP) are being proposed regularly, often taking credit for what has been around for decades. I have just read one such book. Many ideas based on old fashioned ways to improve our memory. This reminded me that in my teens, again very many decades ago, I bought one of my first books, *How to Develop a Super Power Memory* by Harry Lorraine.

I can still recall how, even in those days, he suggested that we remember better by using all of our senses. Smell, touch, taste, hear and see it. The more senses you use the easier it is to recall. Make up moving scenes, exaggerated in colour. When meeting someone for the first time It may help to look them in the eye, repeat their name, and offer a handshake. They may also have a certain smell, so you have used three or four of your senses, well done.

My friends know that I can remember telephone numbers. I make up silly pictures and funny stories about them. The crazier they are, the easier it is to remember the number. Do it as soon as they tell you their number, that is if you are not too preoccupied or concerned about what they are thinking of you and what kind of impression you are making.

How do I do it? Firstly, dismiss any common starting numbers for your area. In our village almost all numbers begin with 30 so I dismiss the 30 as most people have that, only those who came later into the village have 39.

My first village telephone number I learned was Jo Bloggs. Remember 60; husband a policeman so PC49 – 2 so 47 so 306047.

Susan next, same number except she is the one (61 not 60) so 306147.

Donald's sounded like 1066 so I added 9 (9 years older than me) so 301075.

Beryl, has a front garden fence with a low curve 9118 so 309118.

Bill, 44, Manchester City beat Manchester United 8 – 2, so 304482. I guess you guessed I am a City fan, he is United.

Paul, 53 the number of the bus I went on to school, remember 06, then 58 the age he looked when I first met him, so 530658.

Joan 7007 looks like a horse, (the number, not the person) she is riding it, with a shirt number 58 on her back, so 700758.

Susan, my birthday date 23 and 51, so 302351.

Pippa, just keeps going up and repeating itself. We had her and five guests on Christmas day so, 07788990154.

Monica a can-can girl 25 when married John now 61 so 302561.

Lulu and partner were 19 and 18 age they met at university in Brighton so 301918.

There are lots and lots more who all have a story. Look at some of your friends' numbers what comes to mind for you? I am sure that you are saying what a load of rubbish it would be easier to just remember the number in the first place.

As we age, our memory sometimes seems to get worse. But it doesn't have to, you can keep your memory sharp at any age, and improve it at any time. Try.

"Thinking about Thinking"
Higher Reasoning
Executive Function

Prefrontal Cortex

9 Functions of the Prefrontal Cortex

1. Empathy
2. Insight
3. Response Flexibility
4. Emotion Regulation
5. Body Regulation
6. Morality
7. Intuition
8. Attuned Communication
9. Fear Modulation

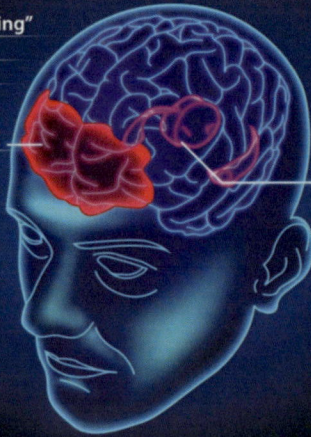

Limbic Brain

1. Fight, flight, freeze stress response
2. Thinks, "Am I safe? Do people want me?"
3. Emotions live here

Are You Right-Brained or Left-Brained?

R **L**

Right brain attributes
- Creativity
- Like shapes / patterns
- Singing / music / theater / art
- Visualizations
- Likes to see the "whole" picture
- Emotional
- Colors
- Active
- Prefers essay tests to true / false
- Willing to take risks
- Finds similarities
- Sensitive to thoughts / emotions
- Asks "why" more often than "how"

RIGHT-EARED →

L — RIGHT-EYED

Left brain attributes
- Linear thinking
- Detail / fact oriented
- Reading / phonics / language / talking
- Auditory / listening
- Like the "parts" before the "whole"
- Logical
- Numbers
- Time-oriented
- Prefers true / false to multiple-choice
- Doesn't like to take risks
- Looks for differences
- Prefers things with concrete rules / definitions
- Asks "how" more often than "why"

← LEFT-EARED

R — LEFT-EYED

CONTROLLED BY THE **LEFT BRAIN**
CONTROLLED BY THE **RIGHT BRAIN**

How to find your dominant brain

1. Circle the **EAR** that you would use to listen through a door.
2. Circle which **EYE** is stronger (see guide).
3. Circle the **HAND** that you would use to write or eat.
4. Circle the **FOOT** you would use to kick a ball.
5. Count all circled **L's** and **R's.**

L — RIGHT-HANDED
R — LEFT-HANDED
L — RIGHT-FOOTED
R — LEFT-FOOTED

How to find your stronger eye

1. Extend your arms and make a triangle with your thumbs and forefingers.
2. Center a light switch in the triangle.
3. Close each eye.
4. Which one keeps the switch centred? That's your stronger eye!

Mostly L's = Right brained. **Mostly R's** = Left brained. **Equal L's and R's** = Balanced brain!

WWW.THEPREMIERTUTORS.ORG

4. You Cannot NOT Communicate

Communicating

So, let us begin with the fact that – You cannot NOT communicate.

You only get one chance to make a first impression.

Most first meetings may begin with a handshake. How easy do you find shaking hands?

Communication is two ways. We take in 55% of our communication by body language. When you are saying nothing, you are saying so much, often unaware of what you are indicating to others.

Think of someone that makes you feel good without their speaking. Yes, the smile, the wave, the hug or the warm handshake. Most people are aware of these gestures as being friendly, caring and loving. However, what about that handshake, have you ever asked for, or been given, feedback on how you shake hands? Is it like a droopy wet fish, an iron grip that leaves ring marks in the skin, a simultaneous patronising tap on the back of the hand, or is it a warm genuine gesture?

Ask someone you trust to give you feedback.

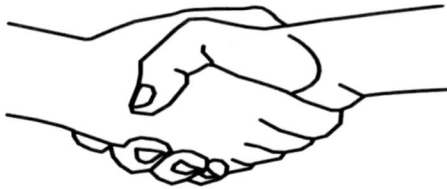

Now think of the person that makes you feel criticised, unworthy, even threatened or angry. I bet they point their finger at you. No matter how positive the words are, if you are pointing your finger at someone, it makes them feel negative. You are psychologically coming from the ego state of critical parent.

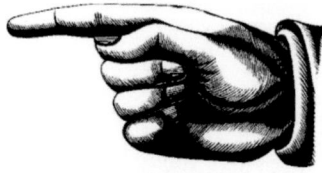

Confucius said, "When you point one finger at someone, you are pointing three back at yourself!"

If you are shaking hands, then do so with your hand as far up to the other person's thumb as you possibly can. Shake firmly, for there is nothing worse than a limp, wet-trout handshake. Equally, it is just as off-putting if you shake hands with a vice-like grip that almost cuts rings into your victim's fingers OR you may be shy or extra strong and aggressive.

You never get a second chance to make a first impression, so give a positive handshake.

5. Body Language

In terms of your body language, you are likely to be aware that certain body positions can trigger certain perceptions in other people's minds. Although you may not really think it matters, you are wrong – it does. It is not what messages you think you are sending, but what is actually being received. "It's not what you say, it's the way that you say it."

Possible feelings or thoughts exhibited:

Body talk (Negative impression transmitted):

Folded arms – Uncomfortable: don't want to be here

Crossed legs – Keep your distance

Turned-up foot – Uncomfortable with what you are saying or what is being asked of you

Arms behind the head – One day you'll be as intelligent as I am, *or* open and too relaxed to be taking this meeting seriously

Hands above shoulders – De-powering, also when hands are on the face

Fingers over lips – Censoring, concerned about what is being said

Twirling hair – Anxious, childish, nervous (some think it is sexy)

Pointed finger – Accusative, critical

Twitching leg, heel or finger tapping – Stressed, wish to hurry, not really interested or say 'I always do that'

In communication we take in 7% of what we hear of what people are actually saying, 38% of what we see and 55% body language. You may be doing this unconsciously, but nevertheless it is affecting how you are thinking or feeling about that person. For example, saying something positive to someone, but also pointing your finger, will be picked up as criticism rather than praise.

Also remember there are cultural differences in different parts of the world. Some of the gestures I refer to are multi-cultural, others may belong just to the western world.

For example, in the western world, looking into people's eyes when they are talking to you creates the impression that you are listening, whereas in other cultures this may be seen as disrespectful. Similarly, people of different nationalities may have different personal spaces. Some people will naturally move very close to the person to whom they are speaking, whereas in other countries this may not be regarded as acceptable behaviour.

So how do different parts of the body talk to us? Hello! What is your body saying?

Head Talk

The nodding of the head almost universally indicates 'yes', or agreement, whereas the shaking of the head implies the opposite, that is, refusing or disagreeing.

When people are happy, they smile: when they are miserable, they frown or grimace. Most people do both, but some do more of one than the other.

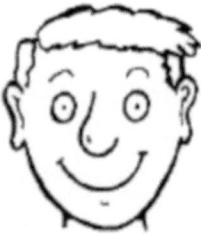

Who do you know who is more likely to smile than look glum?

Whilst the raising of the forehead might be amazement, the raising of eyebrows may indicate puzzlement or disbelief.

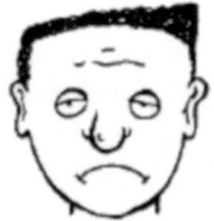

Face Talk

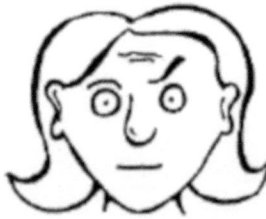

It is not only the movements of the face but also the movements of the hands on the face that indicate when somebody is lying or concerned whether to say anything or not: The hand across the mouth and the finger on the lip may perhaps indicate not wanting to disclose something, censoring.

Lifting the hands above the shoulders and fiddling with hair can disempower you … you are likely to come across as scatty, unsure, or nervous. Some may think it is sexy! Stroking a beard can depower you, or sucking your glasses may again take away your power. The sucking of glasses is also supposed to indicate that you are waiting for time or 'thinking it over' OR it could mean that you are trying to stop smoking and need some oral gratification of the associated breast!

Eye Talk

In neuro-linguistic terms, it is thought that people will move their eyes in different directions depending on what they are seeing, hearing or feeling. These pictures are mirror images of their eyes as you are looking at them. As they raise their eyes to their left (to the right as you look at them) they are trying to recall incidents … To the left, they are creating visually or constructing images.

Looking straight at you means they are listening and slightly to the right shows they are recalling and remembering what they or you have said.

However, when the eyes are lowered it means that people are influenced by kinaesthetic, emotions or feelings; lowered and slightly to the left indicates feelings; and to the right, talking to oneself.

Of course, some people could still be listening to you with their eyes lowered, because what is being said between you is creating a set of positive or negative emotions. Also, some will close their eyes when they are trying to see something, or want to withhold their feelings.

The raising of the eyes to the left or to the right are reversed by six percent of the population. Many of the people in this group are left-handed, but not all. So, in some instances, the eyes move in the opposite direction for recalling and creating to that which has been described.

If you ask someone "What have been your successes over the last year?", they are likely to recall the images visually.

Which way will their eyes go?

When you ask "Where do you see yourself in two years' time?", they are likely to construct the image visually.

Which way will their eyes go?

"What do you think you will say to her at your next meeting?"

Auditory construct. Which way will their eyes go?

"How do you feel about not getting your promotion?"

A kinaesthetic response. Which way will their eyes go?

"What might you say to yourself before your next demonstration?"

Leads to an auditory dialogue. Which way will their eyes go? Try using this information next time you are interviewing or are talking with someone where you want to know the truth.

Shoulder Talk

The shoulder shrug is usually accepted as meaning "I don't quite understand:" "I don't care:" "I don't really know what you are talking about", whereas if the shoulders are lifted, with tension around them, this may indicate fear.

We lodge fear in our shoulders, anger in our calves and, supposedly, sexual dysfunction in the lower back! OR you could have just slipped a disc or pulled a muscle! If your arms are folded, this can indicate that you want to block somebody out or, more likely, that you are feeling uncomfortable with yourself or the situation you are in.

Many people will say "I only cross my arms like this because it makes me feel more comfortable", and they are right, because when we are feeling uncomfortable inside, we give ourselves a little cuddle. OR you may be cold, be trying to hide your bitten fingernails, even wishing to cover your chest!

Touch Talk

A lot of information can be gleaned from touch. The most likely tactile interaction in people management is probably going to be the handshake. This is so important when meeting colleagues, or new clients, for the first time. In terms of hands, you can have a submissive hand, where the palm is uppermost, or a dominant hand, where the palm is lowered. Shaking hands can create a tremendous impression, good or bad, on your first meeting with someone.

If you are shaking hands, then do so with your hand as far up to the other person's thumb as you possibly can. Shake firmly, for there is nothing worse than a limp, wet-trout handshake.

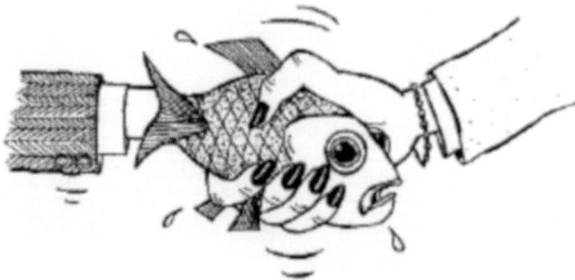

Equally, it is just as off-putting if you shake hands with a vice-like grip that almost cuts rings into your victim's fingers.

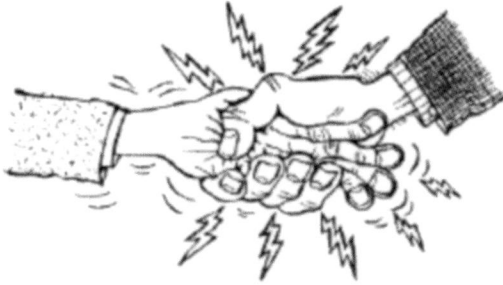

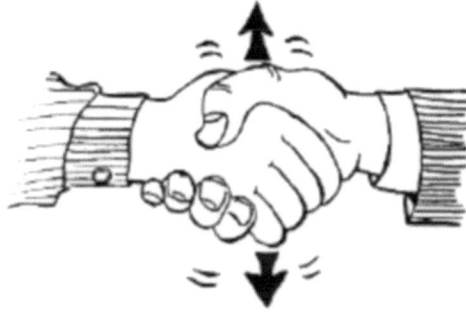

Statements like 'shake like a man' are often indicators of firmness and power. However, whether male or female, you need to shake someone's hand firmly but not tightly.

Then there is the gloved handshake, where someone will put both their hands around yours, shaking with one hand and covering the back of your palm with the other. This may make people feel smothered, patronised or even intimidated.

In some countries people may hold your elbow, wrist, upper arm or even your shoulder while shaking your hand. It has been said that culturally they may be feeling up the arm for a hidden weapon.

Hand Talk

If somebody is sitting with their elbows on the table and their intertwined fingers, blocking their body, this may indicate a tendency to hold in negative feelings, even though they may be smiling. Intertwined fingers indicate resistance, whereas open hands show acceptance. OR you may be tired and need to lean on your elbows.

The higher the hands are held, the more resistant the person is likely to be, although clenched hands held low down the body would still tend to keep people at bay.

Then there is the 'steepling' of hands. The 'raised steeple' indicates someone who thinks in terms of superiors and subordinates (awful words!). So it gives the impression of interacting as a superior talking to a subordinate. A kind of know-it-all or confident attitude. Teacher managers often use this gesture when they want to give advice to their subordinates. However, you may have noticed that many management books and managers use this word 'subordinate' instead of 'colleagues' or 'staff'.

The 'lowered steeple' indicates that you are listening rather than feeling in control and superior. OR that you are protecting your vulnerable areas!

Body Talk

Does my body language give me away?

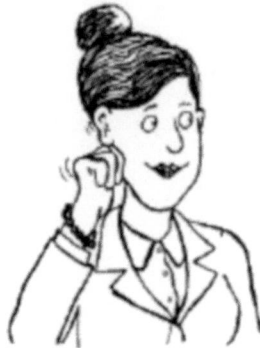

It is important to give positive rather than negative messages to the people with whom you associate. So, let us now look in detail at how your body can talk. What it might say even though you may not mean to be giving out such a message.

Never underestimate the power of your body language. How you use your body almost certainly affects people and how they may react or feel about you. It is, however, an area that is often dismissed as psychological gobbledegook, or there is a reluctance to accept its relevance.

When someone talks to you, you are only hearing seven percent of

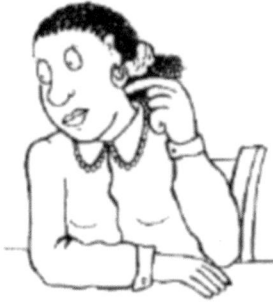

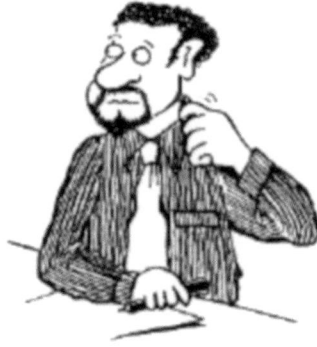

Eye Talk

In neuro-linguistic terms it is thought that people will move their eyes in different directions depending on what they are seeing, hearing or feeling. These pictures are mirror images of their eyes as you are looking at them. As they raise their eyes to their left (to the right as you look at them) they are trying to recall incidents …

Eye movement sketches needed here

To the left, they are creating visually or constructing images. Looking straight at you means they are listening and slightly to the right shows they are recalling and remembering what they or you have said.

However, when the eyes are lowered it means that people are influenced by kinaesthetic, emotions or feelings; lowered and slightly to the left indicates feelings; and to the right, talking to oneself.

Matters, you are wrong – it does. It is not what messages you think you are sending, but what is actually being received. "It's not what you say, it's the way that you say it."

So test it out. Begin by looking at the following illustrations and write down what you would feel or think about a person if they were to use such a gesture.

Some people may find this difficult and respond with, "Nothing – I'm not affected by body language. I don't stereotype people."

Well, good for you, but I believe that you will be affected subconsciously, if not consciously, by how people use their bodies.

So many teachers, with whom I have worked as a trainer, have initially laughed at the idea, only to be convinced of its importance. Usually this happens because they have received feedback from other delegates on the same course about their negative perceptions of the cynic's body language.

So, fake it till you make it
Ten tips on body language in interviews

1. Shake hands firmly, not aggressively
2. Smile only when genuinely pleased
3. Keep arms below shoulders
4. Keep legs un-crossed
5. Put feet firmly on floor
6. Keep arms open
7. Keep hands relaxed
8. Have open, accepting body posture
9. Keep still: stillness is empowering
10. Hold your head at the same angle as the interviewee

5b. Projection

Apart from our communicating non verbally, without realising what others are picking up about us, we also reveal many things about ourselves in speech.

We say much more about ourselves when we are talking about others, than we ever say about the named person to whom we are addressing, referring to, writing about, and talking about, complementing or criticising. Numerous times you hear some people project their *own* inadequacies, opinions, values, behaviour and fears on to others. This is called projection. It means that you very often witness some diabolical insult or description of someone, only to find yourself thinking 'That sounds more like you than the person to whom you are referring, lambarding, humiliating or describing.

According to Karen R. Koenig, M. Ed, LCSW, projection refers to unconsciously taking unwanted emotions or traits you *do not* like about yourself and attributing them to someone else.

Carl Jung said that Hitler was a mad man but Hitler accused Churchill of being a madman and running around Europe starting fires and telling lies. Projection of his own behaviour. Here we are today witnessing the same behaviour of projection with different names Putin and his projection on to Zielinska.

A more frequent common example of projection is a cheating partner who suspects and accuses their partner of being unfaithful.

The following Easter article was written by Anna Roberts in the Argus 3rd April 2013 which demonstrates projection.

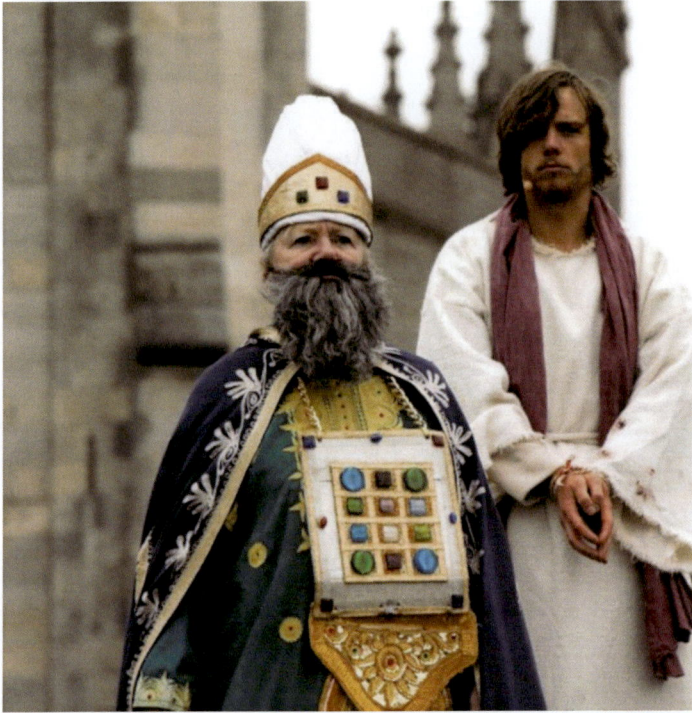

Brighton actress attacked during 'crucifixion' of Jesus

A beard-wearing woman was attacked, as she crucified Jesus.

The crime of Passion took place as the woman played a priest during the open air retelling of the Easter story.

Jeanie Civil's attacker ripped her beard from her face and punched her during a performance of The Passion of Christ in Brighton on Easter Sunday, 2013.

He yelled "Shame on you!" before Mrs Civil's fellow cast members, dressed as soldiers, held him back. He was bundled into a police car.

About 1,000 people were watching Mrs Civil playing Joseph Caiaphas in the grounds of St Peter's Church when the man jumped up and attacked.

Yesterday Mrs Civil said: "He was hooded. He leapt up and punched me. He then pulled my beard from my face. It really hurt and it was very shocking." Mrs Civil – a psychologist, psychotherapist and author – said she wondered if the man was an ardent Christian who disliked her character's actions towards the saviour.

In the New Testament, Caiaphas was the Roman-appointed Jewish high priest who is said to have organised the plot to kill Jesus. According to the

Gospel, Caiaphas was the major antagonist of Jesus and was involved in the trial of Jesus.

Mrs Civil, who is from Ovingdean, said: "I was walking down the side. He jumped up and hit me. I had to stop him hitting me again. He might be an ardent Christian, or anti-Jewish. If he has mental health problems then I really hope he gets support." She said she carried on acting but had to hold her beard to her face. A Sussex Police spokesperson said: "A man was arrested on suspicion of assault at around 4pm on Easter Sunday."

"The assault took place during a performance outside St Peter's Church in York Place, Brighton, on a female member of the cast. A 59-year-old Brighton man was arrested on suspicion of assault by beating and has been bailed until May 1, pending further enquiries."

It turned out at his court case in Brighton that he had been fighting in Afghanistan and had recently been released from there, he felt great anger towards men who looked like me and was very hurt by those exercised such power and influence over the crowd of a thousand outside St Peters, to convince them to kill Jesus and release Barabbas.

He was an alcoholic, and he was given a 6-month suspended sentence, if he attended alcoholics anonymous and was given mental health support.

He later sent me a message saying he was so sorry to have hurt me.

6. Everyday Counselling

Everyone has difficult experiences, both at work and at home. By using counselling skills, you can enable other people to deal with their concerns, making it easier for them to work through their feelings.

An essential counselling skill is to give time and space for people to handle their experiences. These experiences may usually leave people with a sense of loss; not only bereavement but other experiences too, like parents' break up, exam failure loss of expected promotion or broken relationships. By giving time to other people you can help them to change a painful experience into a painful memory.

Every day counselling is what almost all of us do from time to time for friends and colleagues. Friendship certainly helps, but acquiring specific basic counselling skills and also knowing the pitfalls to avoid will most certainly assist the person needing support.

How to Start

Offer a warm, friendly, non-judgemental, genuine relationship and you will be supporting someone effectively.

Body Language

An open posture shows the other person that you are really listening, it will also help you as well. Try to keep still, with your arms and legs uncrossed, feet on the floor and with your hands relaxed. This will help the other person to feel that you are listening and concentrating on them alone. It is quite hard to achieve this and it takes practice as there is a natural tendency to interrupt and contribute to the conversation.

Watch out for signs that the other person is feeling uncomfortable. The position of their feet or arms can sometimes indicate this. People may turn up their toes, or cross their arms or legs creating a 'barrier'.

Active Listening

One of the most important practical skills is active listening. That means listening with your ears, eyes, heart and brain. Then summarise what you have heard. Do this on two levels, firstly what the person has said and what you have understood. Secondly what they have not said but what you have heard.

You may decide to keep that observation to yourself and check it out later. Give good non-verbal feedback by your displaying what you now known as open body language.

Reflect Back

What you have heard by describing what you think the person is trying to tell you. Avoid hurrying or giving solutions. An important skill is to ask open questions (that means questions that cannot be answered with a one-word answer like 'yes' or 'no').

Ask *how* and *what* questions not *why* because why is threatening.

Which question is less threatening:

Why were you late? or

What happened to make you late?

'Why do you feel like this?' or

'What has happened to make you feel like this?'

Listen to the *music* behind the words

Listen with your *third* ear

Hear with your *eyes* and see with your *ears*

Listen to the *feeling* as well as the story

Generation / Value Gap

We all have different values, attitudes, cultures, religions and feelings. A person may come to you because of your values or because you have the same religion, culture, sexual orientation, race or gender or because they respect your age or attitudes.

Many people think that they have been given good advice when they hear what they want to hear. When someone asks you, "What would you do if you were me?" Try answering, "I wonder what you would like me to say?" The person may then tell you with their answer what the solution is to their own inner conflict, e.g. "I want you to say (resign, leave him/her, don't do it, say sorry, keep your money, go on holiday, move house, change your mind, save your marriage, stop feeling guilty, buy it, it's not your fault, be happy, wait and see what happens, stop the affair right now, adopt, keep it a secret. you are right.) …"

See the World through Their Eyes

Empathise; this means trying to see their world through the other person's eyes; listen through their ears; walk in their shoes; feel through their experience; think through their frame of reference.

Give people the opportunity to show their emotions. Give them permission to feel; permission to grieve; permission to be angry and – equally important – permission to be happy.

So try to avoid using the standard phrases in a way that makes the person feel that their emotions are unacceptable. Saying "I know how you feel" is untrue and unhelpful.

Understanding and using emotions is recognised as being essential to thinking, being creative and solving problems.

We have two brains, the feeling brain and the thinking brain. The feeling brain is even more powerful than the thinking brain. When we are upset the thinking brain shuts down.

Have you ever heard someone say, "I can't think straight right now as I am too emotionally upset."?

Try to join the person where they are at the time. Accept how they feel and just listen. Avoid trying to suggest a solution. Often there is no solution but the person will feel much better if they think and feel that you have listened to what they have said.

Their Story, not Yours

Silence is often more helpful than words. When a person comes to you with some issue or concern, they need to talk about themselves, their feelings, and their experiences. They do not want to hear about what has happened to you in your life. Manners, stops them from talking whilst they have to listen to your often-indulgent reminiscences. I know you will think *rubbish I do it to help them*.

No two experiences are the same. Whilst the situation may be similar in its nature, it can never be identical; so, do not join in with your own reminiscences. If you go to see a doctor about your operation scar, you do not expect them to roll up their vest and show you their scars, do you? So, as their friend or colleague don't reveal your emotional scars.

You may think it will help and it is for them, but 99% of disclosures are for the discloser! So, a word of warning don't share what happened to you, the fact that you need to talk about yourself can mean that you have unfinished business and shows a lack of empathy towards the other person.

You can empathise without having experienced the same story. What feeling words are they using? Betrayed, hurt, embarrassed, lonely, jealous, angry, guilty, happy or relieved. You may not have had the same thing happen to you but it is highly likely that you have felt the same feelings with a different story of your own.

Counselling Tips what do you remember?

Your body language – keep arms and legs uncrossed, feet on the floor and hands loose.

Create rapport – by mirroring both the other person's body and their language.

Active listening – that is listening with your ears, eyes, heart and brain and reflecting (summarising) what you have heard them say, as well as being aware of what they have not said. Use silence.

Asking open questions – using 'what' and 'how' but respect the person's right to say, "No, that's enough for today."

Go at their pace – seeing through their eyes, listening through their ears, walking in their shoes. Avoid digging and delving.

Zipping up – by getting them to set their own targets or changes, then checking out their feelings about the time with you.

Taking responsibility

Work towards the person being able to take responsibility for themselves. Whilst it is good to be supportive, it can exacerbate the situation, if you try to do everything for them. Ask them what they think that they can achieve and then get them to set out how they think that they can achieve their chosen targets.

Go for small successes not big failures.

Boundaries

Counselling and friendship are different. When you act as an everyday counsellor (even if you are also a friend) you need to create boundaries that stop you from becoming involved in someone's private life.

Touch

We can say so much more by touching than we can with words. It is a pity that people are losing out on the warmth and genuine love which results from appropriate touch but it must be for the other person, not you, to decide if touch is appropriate. Ask permission. Be genuine not a phoney. There are appropriate places to touch like shoulders. I am often moved to quickly touch a hand or knee when someone is very distressed.

Pitfalls in Counselling

We may feel anxious when people come to see us and wonder if we can meet their expectations. These feelings may cause us to act in some of the following named behaviour types:

Mr Busy – Being too busy to listen. Too busy – not making time for people.

Mrs Psychoplonker – Some individuals fancy themselves as a psychologist or psychiatrist.

Mr Nosey – Asking too many irrelevant questions. Talking too much.

Mr Chatterbox – Being unable to cope with silence. Having to fill the silence.

Mr Gruesome Twosome – Wanting to be 'intimate' with the person that you are supporting. Agreeing and condoning maybe some illegal or inappropriate behaviour in order to be liked and feel accepted.

Mr Me – Identifying with the person, but imposing our own experiences. Identifying too closely

Mr Prejudice – Threatened by different cultures, religions, politics or gender. Considering own needs not the other persons.

Mrs Oldie – Feeling threatened by the generation gap. Too keen to provide a quick fix. Not allowing the person to express their needs.

Mrs Don't Delve – Finding a quick solution, which only deals with the present problem.

Mr Fix-It – Wanting to do everything for the person.

Mr Blocker – Blocking the other person's emotions.

Ms Moral – Dictating and imposing our values onto the individual.

Professional Help Everyday counselling by friends and colleagues can provide a much-needed help and support, however some people will need professional help. If someone appears to need more help or if you feel 'out of your depth', you can help the person to acknowledge that they need professional guidance.

Information about professional counselling can be obtained by consulting a GP or the British Association for Counselling and Psychotherapy.

(Tel 0870 443 5252) email: bacp@bacp.co.uk

If you want to talk confidentially to someone that you feel that you can trust you can always telephone Samaritans and it is free.

7. Caring

In the last 40 years, evolutionary psychological research has focused on the pursuit of love and sexual partners and its effect on their behaviour but according to the latest results of a global study published in *Perspectives in Psychological Science*, most people believe that caring for their family members is their top priority and rated the former as the least important factor in their lives.

In our present global world virus crisis this will resonate for so many of us.

An international team of researchers led by evolutionary and social psychologists from Arizona State University (ASU) surveyed 7,000 people from 27 countries about what matters most to them.

The results of the research demonstrated that people who rank mate-seeking as their most important objective were less satisfied with their lives and were more likely to be depressed or anxious. Whilst people who rated family care and long-term relationships as the most important features of their lives reported the highest sense of well-being.

These findings were then replicated in different cultures like collectivist cultures, e.g. South Korea and China, and in individualistic cultures, like Europe and the United States.

"Studying attraction is easy and sexy, but people's everyday interests are actually more focused on something more wholesome—family values," said APS Fellow Douglas Kenrick, an ASU psychological scientist and senior author on the study. "Everybody cares about their family and loved ones the most, which, surprisingly, hasn't been as carefully studied as a motivator of human behaviour."

"People might think they will be happy with numerous sexual partners," Kenrick said, "but really they are happiest taking care of the people they already have." So maybe all that toilet paper, we were witnessing being grabbed, in the pandemic was for the whole family.

8. Emotions Have Intelligence!

Traditionally in our western society, we associate intelligence with thinking, remembering, analysing, comparing, applying, examinations and grades. Many of us spend a lot of time developing our thinking skills. Our feelings, our emotions are mainly ignored. The concept of emotional intelligence covers a broad collection of individual skills generally referred to as inter and intra-personal skills that are outside the traditional areas of specific knowledge, general intelligence and technical or professional skills.

Current thinking on the topic maintains that in order to be a well-adjusted, fully functioning member of society, family member, a partner, employee or friend we need to possess both Traditional Intelligence (IQ) and Emotional Intelligence (called EQ).

What does it mean? EQ means being empathic, putting our self in the other person's frame of reference, listening through their ears, seeing through their eyes, walking in their shoes and feeling with their heart.

Emotional intelligence can be learned. That is why older people are more likely to have a higher EQ. Mainly because they have learned to recognise how others are affected by their behaviour. Perhaps they have unintentionally hurt them with a passing remark.

Also, with age they will also have experienced numerous personal and emotional situations in their own lives.

Empathy is essential in EQ. However, do we need to recognise if we need to, always show empathy, all of the time, or are there times when it is inappropriate?

Racist remarks for instance.

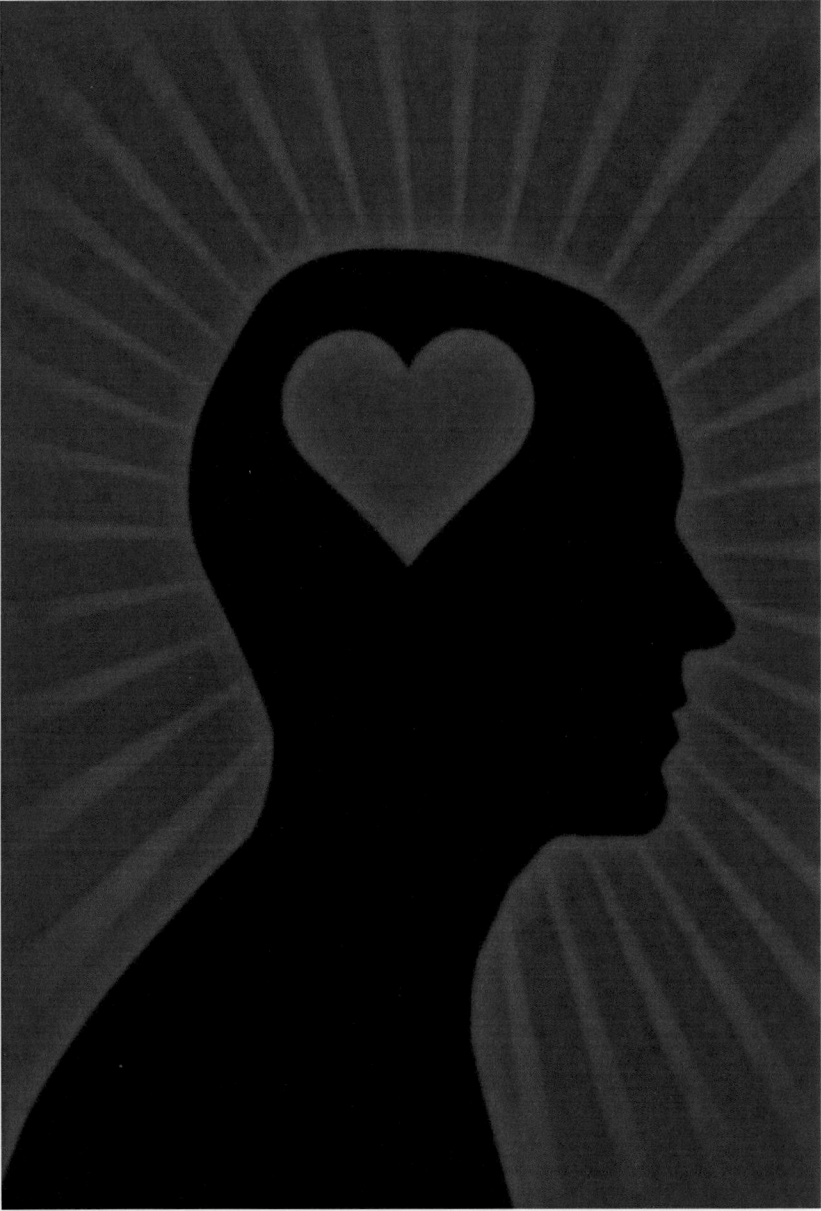

9. Giving Feedback with Love

GIVING COMPLIMENTS (Called Warm Fuzzies)

DISCOUNTING COMPLIMENTS (Called Cold Prickleis)

We have a chuff button and we have a crumple button. Warm fuzzies, compliments, make us feel warm and happy all over, whereas 'cold prickleis' hurt and make us feel uncomfortable. Being able to give and receive compliments without embarrassment or denial reflects a healthy level of self-worth. How mentally healthy are you in giving and receiving compliments?

Look at the scenarios below. Note your most likely response.

1.   Your manager compliments you on a report you have prepared. What do you think or do?

   a)   Reply "Thanks, but I don't really think it's that good."
   b)   "Thank you, that feels good."
   c)   Think to yourself "What are you after?"

2.   David, a junior member in your team, has just delivered an excellent presentation to one of your clients. What do you think or do?

   a)   Think to yourself "Keep your hands off! This one's mine!"
   b)   Oh well, they'll probably want David, not me, to handle their account from now on.
   c)   Walk over and say "Well done, first-rate presentation. I really think it went down well with the client."

3.   You are congratulated on winning promotion. What do you think or do?

    a)   Say, "Thanks! I'm absolutely thrilled!"
    b)   "I should think so too, after all the hard work and time I have put into this company."
    c)   "It was a fluke; I don't really deserve it!"

Ever heard yourself saying to a compliment given to you
"I like your dress!"
"What this old thing? I got it from a charity shop" –
"I like your dress too" or
"I wear it when I feel fat."
Just say thank you!

We discount people by giving the same warm fuzzy back to them.

A cold prickly starts off with a warm fuzzy but ends with criticism
e.g.
You are very intelligent, for a woman or
You are very sensitive, for a man.

Our mental health is enhanced when we believe that we are valued, wanted, loved, appreciated. Who comes into your mind that gives you that warm fuzzy feeling? Try accepting compliments rather than discounting them. Just say thank you and enjoy feeling good.

Mental Health

10. Mental Health

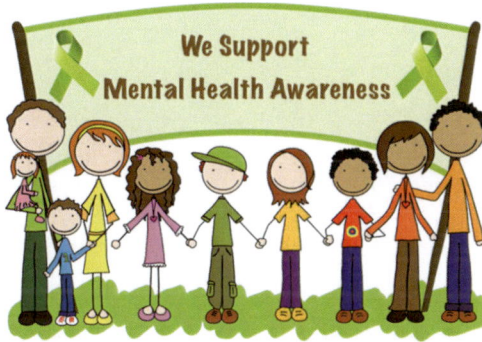

We hear a lot about the increase in mental health or perhaps, it is mental ill heath that is on the rise, and I wonder why. Whilst both men and women, suffer with issues of becoming mentally ill they do not 'suffer' in equal measures.

In England, women are more likely than men to have a common mental health issue and are almost twice as likely to be diagnosed with anxiety disorders. But more men than women commit suicide. In 2013, 6,233 suicides were recorded in the UK for people aged 15 and older. There were 78% male and 22% female. Today's suicide figures are approximately 75% men and 25% female.

10% of mothers and 6% of fathers in the UK have mental health problems at any given time. In the cases of depression, one in ten of us will suffer from depression to some degree or other. What day of the year do you think is the most depressing? Of course, this varies as for many of us it might be the anniversary of a loved one's death or the memorable date of someone leaving us and their children for someone else. Whilst many us may say in answer, New Year's Eve, (a miserable 10 million Britons say New Year's Eve is the 'most depressing' night of the year) or Christmas Day but actually Valentine's Day is higher on the list, but recent research states that the third Monday in January is the most depressive day.

So Valentine's Day has gone and the hope of spring and seeing sunshine and sprouting daffodils brings a smile to most people's faces as we feel the sun's warmth and look at the sea's stillness, if we are lucky enough to ever see the sea.

Mental **health** is much more than a diagnosis. It's your overall psychological well-being—the way you feel about yourself and others. Making changes pays off in all aspects of your life, boosts your mood, builds **resilience**, and adds enjoyment to life: Tell yourself something positive. Research shows that **how you think about yourself** can have a powerful effect on how you feel. One of the people in the village said to me that when she was ill she heard a doctor on the radio saying if you think you are well, you are well. It helped her as it helped me when she told me. **Gratitude** has been clearly linked with improved well-being and mental health, as well as **happiness**. Keep a gratitude journal or write a daily gratitude list. Exercise your body; it releases **stress**-relieving and mood-boosting endorphins before and after you do it. It lessens **anxiety**, and **depression**.

Eat a good, nutritious meal. What you eat nourishes your whole body, including your brain.

Open up to someone. Knowing you are valued by others is important for helping you think more positively about yourself. Plus, being more trusting can increase your emotional well-being because as you get better at finding the positive aspects in other people, you become better at recognising your own.

Do something for someone else. It has a beneficial effect on how you feel about yourself and is a great way to build your **self-esteem.**

Take a break. Take a deep breath, step away, and do anything but what was stressing you.

Go to bed earlier. Sleep deprivation has a significant negative effect on your mental health and mood.

11. Depression (Painful Emotions)

I am fed up, I am cheesed off, I have nothing to look forward to, nothing goes right in my life, I am lonely, I don't have any friends, nobody rings me, nobody loves me, I am an outsider, I am depressed, I am mentally ill, I have been diagnosed as clinically depressed, I feel suicidal.

Have you ever thought or felt any of these statements or found yourself in these situations?

What a range of emotions, from feeling fed up to suicidal, such a spectrum of words are often used under the umbrella of feeling depressed.

Yes, depression does affect your mood, thoughts, feelings, behaviours and physical health. Whereas severe depression can result in your losing the ability to feel pleasure in the things that you once enjoyed. It can also mean that you want to withdraw from your social relationships even from people with whom you are closest.

(17 Dec 2020) The enforced separation of families and friends in the pandemic, will no doubt in the future, when figures are analysed, will show to have increased peoples' depression.

While Freud (1917) proposed that many of the cases of depression were due to biological factors, it was thought in the sixties that a deficiency of noradrenalin in certain parts of the brain was responsible for creating a depressed mood.

Whereas now, in the 2020s, there is growing evidence that several parts of the brain shrink (where there is a lot of brain cells) in people with depression. The evidence shows that the loss seems to be higher in people who have regular or ongoing depression with serious symptoms.

Freud also argued that some cases of depression could be linked to the loss of or rejection of a parent, as well as childhood abuse, be it physical or mental.

Today there is great deal of evidence to show how sexually abused children are highly likely to suffer from depression as an adult, and the new law changes have shown how mental abuse leading to depression can be defensive evidence in murder cases.

There are different types and degrees of depression, but it is hardly everyday psychology;

Major Depressive Disorder (MDD),
Persistent Depressive Disorder (PDD),
Bipolar Disorder, Postpartum Depression (PPD),
Premenstrual Dysphonic Disorder (PMDD),
Seasonal Affective Disorder (SAD),
Atypical Depression.

Just as with any type of depression, atypical depression is a serious mental health condition, and is associated with an increased risk of suicide and anxiety disorders. Atypical depression often starts in the teenage years, earlier than other types of depression, and can have a more long-term (chronic) course.

New research (originated in 1989) is studying the depression of hopelessness, which maybe how many are feeling at present. It seems that cherished warm milk and bread helped.

As many of us already know, cognitive stress reactivity and biological stress reactivity contribute independently to symptoms of depression.

Depression doesn't just get in the way of our being happy. It can also interrupt our ability to think. It hampers our attention, memory and decision-making abilities. It can be caused by issues people have in being unable to develop healthy, respectful, or committed loving relationships.

When we celebrate what may have happened to our brains. Well, Oxytocin, the so-called love hormone, activates feelings of trust and attraction between people when it is released in the brain, and it rises in the early stages of romantic love.

Do you feel better when you are with people that you trust and are attracted to, perhaps that is when you release your Oxytocin?

Perhaps you can think of a new word to replace depressed, when you feel like using it, in response to being asked "how are you feeling?"

How do you feel right now? Wanted, excited, happy, peaceful, replete, cherished, needed, belong, healthy, warm, valued, loved? Now say it out loud.

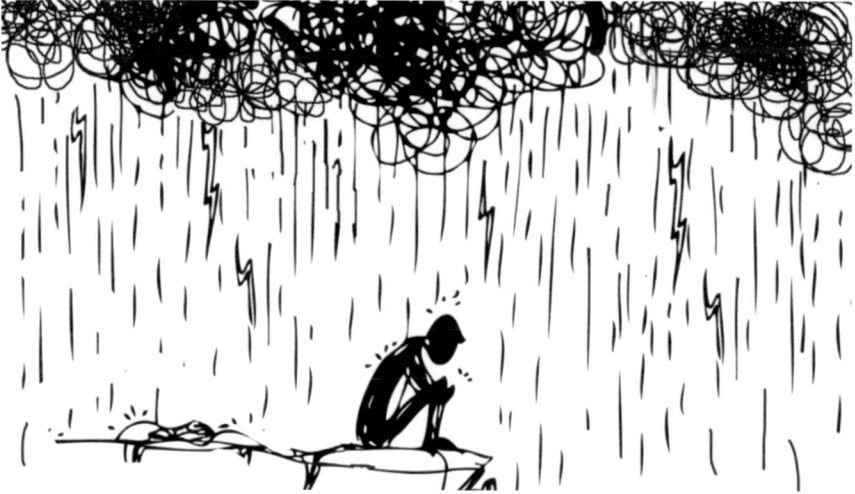

Change your language and you change your feelings.

12. Fear and Phobias

What frightens you?

There is a great deal of fear around at present with the pandemic of Coronavirus.

We are all fearful of very different things. What may frighten one person can seem irrational and pathetic to another. However, the thoughts and physical reactions are often very similar.

How do you tend to handle or react to a stressful fear?

You are likely to be familiar and have heard about our basic human behaviour responses to fear; **freeze**, **fight** or **flight** and are likely to have seen many adverts along these lines.

Fear is a natural, powerful, and primitive human emotion. It is necessary to protect us. Fear involves a universal biochemical response as well as a high individual emotional response.

Fear can also be a symptom of some mental health conditions including panic disorder, social anxiety disorder, phobias, and post-traumatic stress disorder.

So, what does frighten you –

Snakes, Heights, Flying, Death, Failure, Driving, Enclosed Spaces, Needles, Spiders, Water, or the fear of Developing a Disease?

And is it one of over a hundred phobias, if so, what is it called?

Called	Fear of
Atychiphobia.	Failure
Thanatophobia.	Death
Nosophobia.	Developing a disease
Arachnophobia.	Spiders
Vehophobia.	Driving

Claustrophobia.	Enclosed spaces
Acrophobia.	Heights
Aerophobia.	Flying
Trypanophobia.	Needles or Injections
Somniphobia.	Falling asleep
Coulrophobia.	Clowns.
Hylophobia.	Trees
Omphalophobia.	The navel
Nomophobia.	Being without mobile phone coverage
Ombrophobia.	Rain

So, there are only *five basic fears*:

1) Extinction—the fear of annihilation, of ceasing to exist.

2) Mutilation—the fear of losing any part of our precious bodily structure.

3) Loss of Autonomy—the fear of being immobilised, paralysed, restricted, enveloped, overwhelmed.

4) Separation—the fear of abandonment, rejection, and loss of connectedness; of *becoming a non-person*—not wanted, respected, or valued by anyone else. The 'silent treatment', when imposed by a group, can have a devastating effect on its target.

5) Ego-death—the fear of humiliation, shame, or any *loss of integrity of the self*; the fear of the shattering or disintegration of one's constructed sense of lovability, capability, and worthiness.

These can be thought of as forming a simple hierarchy, or 'feararchy':

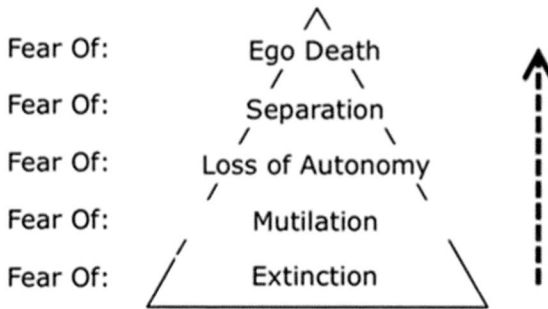

```
                        ∧
Fear Of:            Ego Death            ↑
                    /      \             ┊
Fear Of:           Separation            ┊
                  /        \             ┊
Fear Of:        Loss of Autonomy         ┊
               /           \             ┊
Fear Of:       Mutilation               ┊
            /              \            ┊
Fear Of:  /    Extinction    \          ┊
```

The "Feararchy"

© Karl Albrecht 2007
All Rights Reserved.

President Franklin Roosevelt famously asserted, "The only thing we have to fear, is fear itself."

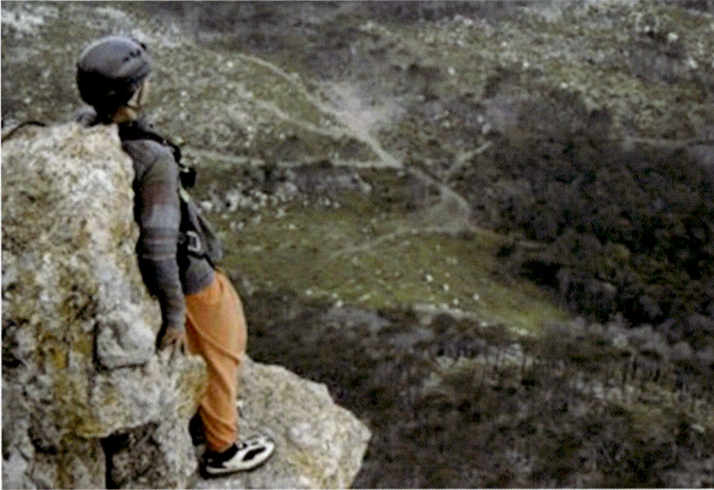

Source: Vitali Nesterchuk/Shutterstock

I think Roosevelt he was right: Fear of fear probably causes more problems in our lives than the fear itself. As fantasy is often worse than reality so mentally we need to be aware of when we are fantasying (making it up) and what is actually true and factual.

Hippopotomonstrosesquippedaliophobia is one of the longest words in the dictionary—and, in an ironic twist, is the name for a fear of long words … (I wonder whatever mental state were the creators, of such a word, in?)

The fear or anxiety is disproportionate to the social situation.

The fear or anxiety is persistent and the social situation is excessively avoided; the thought of having our body's boundaries invaded, or of losing the integrity of any organ, body part, or natural function.

Anxiety about animals, such as bugs, spiders, snakes, and other creepy things arises from fear of mutilation entrapped, imprisoned, smothered, or otherwise controlled by circumstances beyond our control. In physical form, it's commonly known as claustrophobia, but it also extends to our social interactions and relationships.

One way that has a well-known negative mental effect on almost all people is the 'silent treatment' when ignoring you completely is the behaviour you experience. For instance, when you are not involved in an important decision;

56

spoken to any longer; when a group decides to act together to 'get rid of you'. When a group imposes this behaviour, this can have a devastating effect on its target.

Has this ever happened to you, how did you react to those involved and how did you look after yourself? Freeze, fight or flight?

13. Feelings Are Facts

It is vital in your work place, your home or educational, medical, industrial, hospitality or business setting that you remember that feelings are facts.

People are unable to work or to learn when they are emotionally 'churned up' about some issue at work or at home, being bullied, fearful of failure, looking stupid, unattractive, or insecure about home concerns and relationships. They may feel that they are not valued. Maybe their manager is not skilled in giving praise or any kind of feedback. In times of change they may feel that their role in the workplace is unappreciated as it is merged into another department or programme area.

Feelings are facts for children too

From a child's point of view

Feelings are facts when I am in bed and think about my day.

Feelings are facts when my mum and dad argue.

Feelings are facts when the new baby arrived.

Feelings are facts when my dog got lost.

Feelings are facts when granny died.

Feelings are facts when my parents do not like my friends.

Feelings are facts when my parents stop me from staying out late.

Feelings are facts when my brother gets all the attention.

Feelings are facts when my dad left.

Feelings are facts when I am playing.

Feelings are facts when my best friend ignores me.

Feelings are facts when I am left out of being invited to a party.

Feelings are facts when I feel poor.

Feelings are facts when I hear horrible things about my black skin.

Feelings are facts when I am left out of games.

Feelings are facts when my body is changing.

Feelings are facts when I look wrong.

Feelings are facts when I don't know what to do.

Feelings are facts when I feel fat.

Feelings are facts when a boy kissed me.

Feelings are facts when I am physically attracted to somebody.

Feelings are facts in the **classroom.**

Feelings are facts when I feel stupid.

Feelings are facts when I am no good at sport.

Feelings are facts when my teacher doesn't like me.

Feelings are facts when I know the answer but don't like to reply.

Feelings are facts when I think about when I am older.

Feelings are facts when I am bullied.

Our emotions are very powerful. They can make us feel good about ourselves or they can make us feel sad.

How we think affects how we feel.

How we feel affect how we behave.

Understanding our emotions and the emotions of other people is part of what we call emotional intelligence or emotional literacy.

Let us see how you feel as we do a little exercise.

You are lying in bed. You can feel the warmth of your duvet, the comfort of your mattress and the snugness of your pillow around your head.

How are you feeling?

Look around your bedroom.

What can you see that brings back to you good memories?

What can you see in your room that makes you feel a little sad?

What can you see that reminds you of a time when you were small?

Remember, when we think about good things, we have good feelings.

When we think about bad things, we have bad feelings.

What happened to you today?

When you got up this morning how did you, feel?

Try to recall your feelings. Were you excited, unhappy, cross? Use whichever word you want to – describe how you felt.

How long did that feeling last?

Who made you feel good today?

Think of something that you heard today that made you smile?

What have you done today that makes you feel good about yourself?

Has anything happened during the day to upset to you?

Before you go to sleep think about the things that have made you feel really happy today and feel the positive things that people have said to you.

Think of somebody who loves you, who makes you feel like a little Prince or Princess.

Celebrate that lovely feeling.

We will look later at how to deal with people when they upset you. I will show you how to talk to people and tell them how you feel so that you can resolve hurtful situations. Meanwhile visualize this scene with two children

Feelings are facts when granny died

Susan; I am feeling really cold. My granny died in hospital on Sunday.

Stephen; Have you got another granny?

Susan; No, I only had one. I used to have two. I called one granny and one Nana. I liked Granny better than Nana. Nana died when I was five.

Stephen; did you go to the funeral?

Susan; No I didn't. They said I was too young to go to funerals.

Stephen; Do you think you were too young to go to funerals when you were five?

Susan; No course I wasn't too young; I loved her. I do want to go to my granny's funeral but I bet they I can't; Granny used to spend more time with me than either my mum or my dad. She was the one that I used to talk to. I couldn't talk to my mum and dad because they were always too busy working. I loved her such a lot, she made me laugh.

I was sitting on the stairs last night and I heard them talking to some people that I had never seen before and they are going to the funeral and I don't even know who they are. They didn't live with my granny like I did when my mum was in the hospital. I heard my dad say that I couldn't go to the funeral and it's not fair. Grown-ups do not seem to realise that children need to grieve too.

Stephen: I think you should tell them that you want to go. The trouble is that parents sometimes think they're doing the best for you when in fact it isn't the best because they don't bother to ask you how you feel. When you go home from school today tell your dad that you want to go to granny's funeral because you loved her and say they that you want to say your goodbyes to her. It's awful when they die in hospital and you don't get a chance to see them. I suppose your mum thought it was better that you remembered her laughing like she was when she was well, rather than seeing her poorly in a hospital bed.

Susan; Yes, I suppose she might have thought that. I just wish that she had asked me how I was feeling about granny dying. Mum and dad say that they can't cry because they have to be strong for us. I think that is being silly. I think that if you love someone, you will cry. Walking around trying to be Superman and Wonder Woman doesn't help any of us to get over the big empty feeling of loss. My sister's boyfriend said that it is a good thing to cry and that you can't remember the good things about the person until you cry for them. I think he's right. Thanks Stephen I'm going to ask my dad if I can go to the funeral. No I'm not, I'm going to say I want to go to the funeral. I have to go now.

Stephen; Bye then Susan. Remember if you love someone you are going to feel sad if they die but isn't that better than never having had anyone to love you?

Do you know that some people are glad when people die because they want their money? I think crying means you loved them.

Susan; yes I think so too. Bye then see you tomorrow.

14. Emotional Intelligence

"Emotional learning begins in life's earliest moments and continues throughout childhood."

– Daniel Goleman

We started the book by looking back at what happened to us all when we were a child; the scripts we were given, the emotions that we experienced and wondering, maybe even identifying some of the reasons of why today we hold certain thoughts, values and behaviours which may have been affected by those early emotional messages. Some were probably good and helpful whilst others may have been destructive of our present mental health.

Would you describe yourself as emotionally intelligent?

What is Emotional Intelligence?

Emotional Intelligence Is Common Sense.

It is what the experienced, empathic and energised person, parent, teacher, support staff, manager, medic, business worker, scientist may have been doing for decades. They may not have known the language or the theory, however emotional intelligence is what they may have been using.

Your job is easy! Well, it would be, if all you had to do is your job. However, as a working or non-working person, what will make your job very difficult and stressful at times is the fact that you have to deal with and manage emotions; Those of your family, partners, staff, colleagues, managers, friends of course, as well as your own.

You probably spend a disproportionate amount of your time dealing with other peoples' emotions. It is likely that 60% of your psychic energy is used up on this aspect of your work.

Ever since Daniel Goleman's runaway bestseller was published in 1995, Emotional Intelligence has been seen as the neglected attribute, which is key to success in almost all spheres of our lives.

Good teachers and many other leaders are made up of 70% emotional intelligence and 30% of intellectual intelligence. Gorman maintains that good leadership needs 82% emotional intelligence and 18% intellectual intelligence.

Emotional intelligence means that you are 'aware of your feelings', 'what the source is of such an emotion', 'how this then affects your behaviour' and 'how your behaviour affects those around you.'

Being aware of your feelings is not enough because you also need to be able to bridge the gap between you and others in order to communicate those feelings and behaviour.

Hence you may work with people that seem to be highly emotionally intelligent, whilst others may appear to be lacking.

Emotions Have Intelligence!

Traditionally in our western society we associate intelligence with thinking, remembering, analysing, comparing, applying, examinations and grades. Many of us spend a lot of time developing our thinking skills. Our feelings, our emotions are mainly ignored.

The concept of emotional intelligence covers a broad collection of individual skills generally referred to as inter and intra-personal skills that are outside the traditional areas of specific knowledge, general intelligence and technical or professional skills.

Current thinking on the topic maintains that in order to be a well-adjusted, fully-functioning member of society, family member, a partner or an employee we must possess both traditional intelligence (IQ) and emotional intelligence (called EQ).

Thinking Brain and Feeling Brain

We have a thinking brain and feeling brain. The feeling brain is greater than the thinking brain. When we are upset, anxious, or fearful of failing, then the feeling brain takes over and the thinking brain cannot operate to its full potential. Hence you may have heard people saying something like –

"I cannot discuss this right now I am too upset and I can't think straight."

Emotional intelligence recognises that we have intrapersonal skills and interpersonal skills. Being aware of our intra personal skills is recognising what we are feeling and possibly, although not always, why these feelings are happening to us. Some people are very good at one but not necessarily at the other. Hence, someone may be very aware of his or her own emotions but unaware of the other people's feelings. Or they maybe be able to understand how the other person is feeling but not be in touch with his or her own emotions in given situations. Sometimes it is very difficult to be able to even hear what the other person is feeling, if we ourselves are very emotionally 'churned up'.

However just being aware of how we are feeling and empathising with the other person's feelings is not enough. Again, we need to be able to bridge the gap. A person with a high EQ has the competence and interpersonal skills to be able to do this.

Emotional Intelligence Is Not A SOFT Option.

It does not mean that you work in a soft and supportive way the whole time but that you are skilled enough to address difficult situations and difficult interviews with direct, assertive, straight, open, clean and honest interactions. Sometimes we have to make hard decisions and recognise the affects. So we need the skills to address difficult situations like conflict, marginal performance, or discipline.

As well as having the skills and courage to address difficult messages we also need to be able to give feedback of a positive nature for instance in appraisals, giving praise or giving feedback on how effective a colleague has worked. Some people find it very difficult to give or to receive praise, so again these are skills that need to be learned.

Emotional intelligence can be learned. That is why older people are more likely to have a higher EQ. Mainly because they have learned to recognise the affects that the various changes in colleges and education, may have had in the past on students and staff. Also, they are likely to have experienced a long history of different management styles, cultures and college history. With age they will also have experienced numerous personal emotional situations in their home lives.

Empathy is essential in EQ. However, we need to recognise if we need to always show empathy all of the time or are there times when it is inappropriate?

Racist remarks for instance, do we show empathy to someone who holds diametrically opposed views to our own?

Emotions Govern Behaviour!

Emotional intelligence involves being aware of emotions, how they can affect and interact with traditional intelligence and how they impair or enhance our judgement. This ability to monitor our own and others' emotions and use the information to guide our thinking and actions, is generally categorised under the following areas:

* Self-awareness: Observing our self and recognising our feeling as it happens.
* Managing emotions: Realising what is behind our feelings. Hidden agendas maybe
* Behaviour; Finding the best ways to handle our feeling of, fear, anxiety, anger, sadness, with the appropriate behaviour.
* Motivating our self; in order to channel our emotions to achieve our goal.
* Emotional self-control: Delaying the need for immediate gratification and stifling impulses.
* Empathising: Being sensitive to other people's feelings and concerns and taking their perspective. Appreciating the differences in how people feel about things.
* Handling relationships: by being able to manage the emotions of other people and having the social competence, interpersonal and intrapersonal skills to be able to achieve harmony.

Types of Emotion

John Heron has identified a number of types of emotion, which are most commonly 'bottled up' in Western European cultures. They are,

*Anger
*Fear
*Grief
*Embarrassment

You may recognise some of these bottled up in you. These examples may ring bells for you if you ever experienced similar concerns

Anger e.g. "I am angry about the new rota. You know that I asked first for that week's holiday and now I see that Simon has that slot. My wife is furious; she knows the incredible amount of work that I have put into my job but I always overlooked for promotion and never shown any niceness."

Fear e.g. "I hear that some staff will lose their present jobs because of the pandemic and the financial position that we are now in?"

Grief e.g. "My brother died at the weekend and I need Friday off to go to his funeral."

Embarrassment e.g. "Well he kept pressing himself against me, when we were checking the stock in the storeroom. I know I am not imagining it. I felt terrible."

Often, these emotions are intermingled and tied up with other basic human needs; for instance, the need for dignity and self-respect.

This article taken from *Taking Appraisals and Interviews* by Jean Civil ISBN 0 7063 7704 4

You Cannot Not Show Emotions.

Even when you are not speaking, you will be giving off an emotion. When you are trying to support someone and they are demonstrating strong emotions then you might find it difficult to talk to them. There is no magic answer to helping people manage their emotions but the following suggestions may help you to be more effective.

In general, most managers will seek to strike a balance between:

(1) Uncontrolled expression of emotion, by setting boundaries and limits, for example:

* In the time you make available (e.g. "We have one hour.")
* Suppression of feelings is avoided, if, for example:
* Feelings arc identified.
* The manager is empathic.
* In all cases the manager will recognise and accept that:
* No two people deal with life events in the same way.

* The line manager has no right to force their beliefs about emotions and feelings onto the members of staff e.g. "You're wrong, you don't feel hurt."

You may disagree and believe that there are times when you have to impose your beliefs on to staff. Certainly, this may be the case in a disciplinary or competence interview, but not in a supportive interview.

In overall terms, dealing with extreme emotions is assisted when the following points are kept in mind:

1. Emotional release is helpful. Anger turned inwards can result in depression.
2. People need time to recover from an emotional release, so let them know that they are likely to feel shaky or shattered after the session with you. To keep themselves warm.

BEING AWARE OF EMOTIONS

Our Primary Emotions are – Anger, Sadness, Fear, Enjoyment, Love, Surprise, Disgust, and Shame

"People with a greater certainty of EMOTIONAL LITERACY about their feelings, are better Emotional Self-Awareness Pilots of their lives."

– Goleman

Emotional intelligence can be learned. That is why older people are more likely to have a higher EQ. Mainly because they have learned to recognise the affects that the various changes in life, may have had in the past on individuals. Also, they are likely to have experienced a lot of different personality, management styles, cultures, politics, wars and world history. With age they will also have experienced numerous personal emotional situations in their own and others home lives.

Empathy is essential in EQ. however we need to recognise if we need to always show empathy all of the time, or are there times when it is inappropriate?

EMOTIONAL LITERACY is an AWARENESS OF EMOTIONS

15. Domestic Emotional Abuse
(the Archers)

It was written so well. I guess like so many other listeners and therapists, some of the episodes left my questioning the many tale endings until gradually the penny started to drop. As in counselling, we have many bits of the jigsaw before we are able to acquire a fuller gestalt picture. Here are some of my questions and thoughts as I followed the story. What had transpired with his previous wife? What were his true concerns for Helen having to give up working in the shop?

What was so wrong with Helen's hair? What drove Rob to work so deviously to break up Helen's relationships with her best friend Kirsty? What was his motive behind his supposed, casual mention to Helen about her cousin Adam's illicit kiss, was it deeply ingrained homophobia or was it jealousy? Of course, as the story unwinds, new thoughts, is it just another manifestation of his controlling personality? Ah yes, it seems to be just another nail of jealousy and is it his need to control her on every front?

What about his scheming to drive a wedge between Helen and her parents, initiating a new Christmas ritual, that of their being alone? To please him, Helen and Henry had to miss out on the longstanding, warm, loving Christmas arrangements they had always had with Pat and Tony, her mother and father. Rob, categorically, did not want Helen to have any loving relationships. He achieved a split between Helen and her brother Tom and with her friend Ian. Her close friend Kirsty was destroyed by Rob as he lied about her telephone calls, taking delight in badmouthing her. Only Kirsty and Tom were suspicious and wary of him, trying to detect Rob's alternative motives.

What was Rob's real motive for wanting to adopt Henry? Did he really want to be a positive stepfather or was it another intentional lever he was using to split the most precious relationship Helen had, that of loving her son? Children need boundaries and some listeners may have welcomed hearing about 'A bit of discipline does them good.' Maybe some were likely to be thinking *Look at me, I was always hit as a child and it never did me any harm.*

Have you ever wanted to disagree with someone who says that to you? As a therapist, it was inevitable that before Rob's father entered the cast, my thought was clear; he would also be a bully. He was!

So many characters were taken in by his slimey interpersonal transactions. His declared love for Helen and his beseeching of so many of her family and neighbours to recognise her mental illness when she was pregnant and he managed to convince family and friends of how lucky she was to have such a good husband. Even her wise, insightful grandmother, Peggy, gave him several tens of thousands of pounds, trusted him and sang his praises.

His behaviour of constantly nibbling away at Helen's self-worth, resulted in her believing that there was something wrong with her. Until she was finally able to meet and address his ex-wife, Jess. Then she discovered that when she was married to Rob, Jess had also experienced his bullying, controlling, aggressive attitudes and behaviour when she shared her many similar life incidents. Helen left her meeting with Jess, knowing that they had both been victim to his violent sexual behaviour of his habit of demanding penetrative sex against their wishes.

Then came the trial. My thoughts of an old classic, very memorable film of Twelve Just Men with Henry Fonda as the jury foreman, stayed with me throughout the trial. As I recalled how brilliantly the film demonstrated how we make our decisions on our value systems and life experiences. In the film it started with only one man, the foreman Henry Fonda, voting for not guilty, by the end, all twelve agreed. This change of attitude happened as each one recounted their own traumatic experiences, which then resulted in their realisation of their projection of their values on to the accused. The same format was played out in Helen's trial. This time the foreman Nigel Havers initially declared a guilty vote but one woman played the role of Henry Fonda, assisting each of the jury members to recognise that their own experiences and values were what was driving their opinion. What a relief – not guilty.

Today early October, we hear that finally Jazzer, David and Kenton Archer witness Rob attacking Emma Grundy, so as the story goes on I expect some of the people that he was able to convince that Helen was mentally insane might change their minds, we will see but I need to finish the article.

In hindsight of the last few months what remains with me mostly is the anger and regret I feel of how Rob tried to influence hate in Henry towards his mother, as so many separated couples may do to their children, justifiably or not. Also without question was Helen's disclosure of the number of rapes she had had to endure, one of which resulted in the conception of Jack. Tragically she was unable to share this with anybody! It only came out finally in Helen's court evidence, although there had been many hints as to how Rob was behaving sexually. My other sadness was in talking with two local intelligent women, they thought that the story was farfetched and couldn't possibly happen! How wrong they are. Finally let us remember it happens to men also!

I asked a very long-standing friend Judi Geisler to write her thoughts about the story, as someone younger who works with women prisoners and she also chairs a charity that assists women suffering from Domestic abuse in Manchester. Here is her contribution.

"The storyline provoked so many different reactions as I listened to each episode. Initially I felt irritation and annoyance that Rob was treating Helen with so little respect. She was an intelligent and popular woman who was devoted to her young son, Henry.

"As Rob slowly undermined her confidence, my anger grew, not just at him but also at all of her family and friends who were so easily duped by the image carefully created of himself. Why could they not see what he was doing?

"Then his actions became more sinister and I started to feel anxious about his motives for isolating her from everyone who cared about her. Soon I found that I was scared each time I heard his voice. I felt a sense of dread that culminated in real fear as Helen argued with him on that fateful night in their kitchen.

"When she stabbed him I experienced a rush of relief that she had finally found the courage to fight back.

"The subsequent events, including the court case, were extremely well portrayed but for me they now felt like just another radio play.

"On reflection, I know why the programme affected me so deeply. The long and subtle build-up of Rob's control and abuse of Helen rang so true. This is because it was so familiar to so many stories I have heard from women I meet in prisons and at a domestic abuse centre.

"The programme has definitely made many people realise that when this sort of abuse happens, the woman involved is gradually and successfully turned into a helpless object for her abusive partner's purposes. It can and does happen behind so many closed doors in every walk of life."

What a result when the law was changed to take into account how extreme emotional abuse on a person can be the cause and the trigger to cause her to murder her husband. Later with her son's evidence she was released from prison.

I clearly remember thinking that at last justice has been done, and feeling hopeful that other victims would feel encouraged to seek help early on, when I heard that news.

We cannot be mentally healthy and happy in an abusive mental or physical relationship – get help – get out now.

16. Optimism

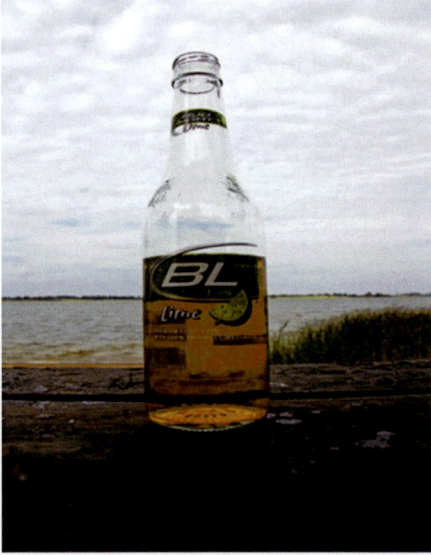

Are you an optimist or a pessimist?

I am sure that you have heard of the psychology behind describing this picture. How do you describe it? Half full or half empty?

Half full is an optimist, half empty is a pessimist. What are your friends and family, are they like you or not?

With a new year coming which way are you going to think? Do you think that how you think can afect how you feel, or how you feel can affect how you think. Of course it can.

Do you feel overloaded by safe tips, suggestons and rules about how to behave and how to feel happier. Well here are some psychological facts.

Positive psychology – is what maximises happiness and well-being rather than dealing with the more negative aspects of human experience.

Buddhism – a range of philosophies that share a belief embracing the inevitable pain and uncertainty of life and regarding suffering is rooted in patterns of craving (people trying to get all what they want and none of what they don't want).

Mindfulness – a range of therapies and self-help practices, drawing on Buddhism, which encourages people to be present with their experiences, paying gentle and curious attention to them, rather than trying to get rid of them or clinging on to them.

Marginalisation – a process of being systematically removed from, and denied participation in, cultural and social activities of a society.

Positive affirmation – positive statements people repeat to themselves, such as "I am a good person".

Stoicism – the idea that people's experience of the world should reflect its nature. People should learn to accept failures, uncertainties and setbacks as part of life, and as part of 'balance' of individual experience.

Rational emotive behaviour therapy (REBT) – a form of cognitive behaviour therapy (CBT) that emphasises shifting people's beliefs in order to alter the impact that adverse circumstances have on them.

Self-help is asking you questions that psychology is best placed to answer about why people have emotional and relationship difficulties. For example, about the best ways of improving thoughts, feelings and behaviours. However, most self-help books are not written by professional psychologists. Research showed that people became happy by changing the ways in which they respond to recognisable negative events. In other words, they have **learned optimistic** ways of responding.

Positive thinking of so much self-help, is an armchair activity, whilst positive psychology on the other hand is tied to a programme of empirical, scientific activity (Seligman 2002). Seligman defines the key elements, positive emotion, engagement, relationships, life's meaning, completing an accomplishment brings mental positivity and positive psychologists do believe that people **can** change how they feel: sad can be transformed into happy. Look at our front cover, these children look optimistic. So almost everybody wants something to which they can look forward.

What are you looking forward to?

17. Hope

We all need hope. As in most chapters I am asking you to just pause for a moment before you read on, and reflect on the topic. So what do you hope for?

Having hope helps us to get through all kinds of mental anxieties. It enables us to think positively about ourselves, our circumstances, our families and friends. It also means that we can take control again of our thought processes. We do not need to be only hopeful of the future, we can actually hope for the now to change for the better by living in today, finding small goals that we can achieve, gives us hope.

Feeling hopeful has many levels from the low expectations of hoping that a film or a book will have a happy ending, or that a chosen menu will taste good, to the deeper hopes, after being hurt by someone. So you may hope when meeting a new partner that this person will lead you into a permanent loving relationship and will take away the existing hurt. Or meeting a new person that you think will be a good foul weather friend only to find that you are mistaken. So you hope again to learn from that rejection and hope that you are able to choose an honest genuine person in the future that will love you. But as Peter used to say "You can't make people love you". So true.

So how many times have you hoped that there is an available car parking space when you go shopping or visiting somewhere for enjoyment; that the new bread is ready when you visit the bakers; the friend who always turns up late this time is going to be on time; that there will still be some super bargain deals left when you arrive late after the crowds. You may hope for financial security; a lot of people hope to solve their monetary issues by winning the lottery; a letter from a loved one or probably most importantly, you may hope for better health.

Like air, we can't live without hope, especially if we're depressed. Why is hope so important? Well when we're excited about 'what's next,' we invest more into our daily life, and we can see challenges. Research shows that unfortunately, only half of us measure high in hope, but fortunately, however, hope can be learned. Hope is not just like optimism it is both the belief in a better future and the action to make it happen.

Hopeful people share four core beliefs that:

1. The future will be better than the present.
2. They have the power to make it so.
3. There are many paths to their goals.
4. They accept that no one is free of obstacles.

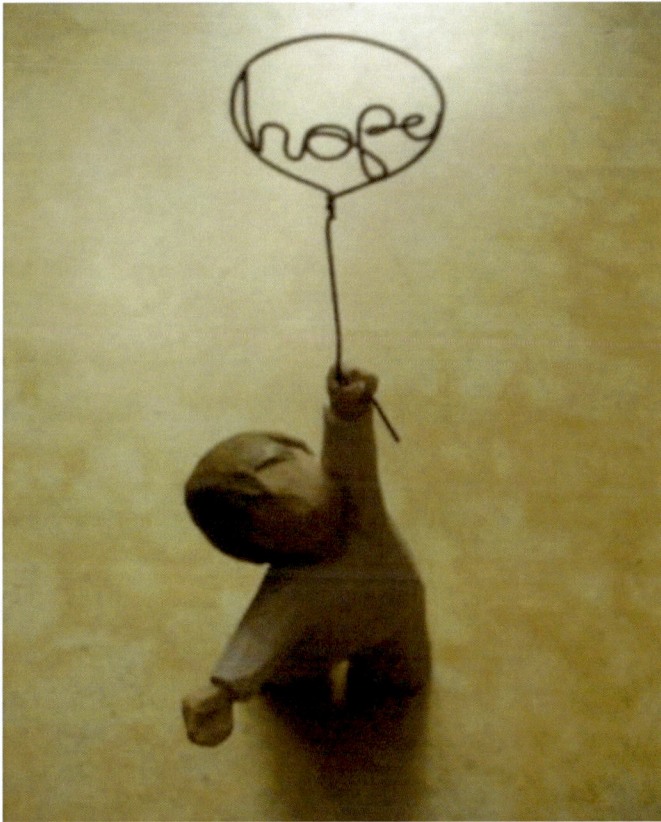

What are your hopes?

18. Belonging

Do you belong? Are you thinking about "to whom do you belong" or "who belongs to you?"

Alternatively, is it in geographical terms, belonging in your, house, your district, your church, your village hall, village club, your hobby, your educational, professional or work group?

Was your first thought, 'I belong to my family'; but what if you have no family?

Celebrating the Kings Coronation this month has raised lots of feelings and thoughts about who belongs to the Royal Family now and who will be included. We now know that Megan and Fergie will not belong to King Charles 3rd's special day.

Our mental health is vital. One of the many things that help us to be mentally well is the feeling that we belong. Our minds have seen us through the pandemic as well as the amazing vaccination programme. The psychology of belonging or love is vital and is one of our major drivers; the need to belong and feel loved. Other motivators for some are to survive, to control, to have money, to have power, to have fun and for many – spirituality. Which is your strongest motivator?

The psyche is the human soul, **mind**, or spirit. The word came (in the mid-17th century) via **Latin** from Greek psukhē 'breathe, life, soul' spirituality. So, as you know psychology is the study of how the mind works. Mental wellness is as vital as physical wellness. Some would say mental wellness is more important than physical wellness.

Belonging is defined as a unique and subjective experience that relates to a yearning for connection with others, the need for positive regard and the desire for interpersonal connection (Carl Rogers, 1951). A sense of belonging does not depend on participation with, or proximity to, others or groups (June 3, 2019).

Many of us are probably yearning for a connection with others but for now, we all need to use other means of creating that feeling of belonging. You could make your own bubble of phone friends, not phoney friends.

Positive psychology experts—those who study human happiness and the factors that contribute to it—have identified several key areas of life that seem to be more related to personal happiness. While it is not an absolute given, that dissatisfaction on one or three areas of life will lead to personal unhappiness or that satisfaction in most areas will automatically lead to bliss, there is a high correlation: if you are more satisfied with these areas of your life, you tend to be happier in general. So, what are the things in life that are correlated with personal happiness? Some of them are the things that you would expect like money, friends, health, living conditions; others are things you may not think of in your daily life, such as your neighbourhood, spirituality, community involvement, and sense of meaning in life. The role that these things play in your life can certainly impact your happiness. How many times have you heard people say that the lock down has made them appreciate their family and the community more?

We have looked at learned optimism and it's probably no secret that optimists tend to be happier people, but you may not realise that there's more to optimism than 'putting on a happy face' or 'looking on the bright side'. There are specific traits of optimists, pleasantly distorted ways of thinking, that do bring optimists more success, greater health, increased life satisfaction, and other perks on a regular basis.

Cultivating the mind of an optimist can not only mean cultivating happiness, regardless of your circumstances, but it can actually bring more things into your life to be happy about.

So, the Psychology of Belonging explores why feeling like we belong is so important throughout our lives, from childhood to old age, irrespective of culture, race, gender or geography.

Part of the grieving process when someone in your life dies, is the loss and emptiness that we feel because we no longer belong to that person, nor them to us.

With its virtues and shortcomings, belonging to groups such as families, social groups, schools, workplaces and communities is fundamental to our identity and wellbeing, even in a time when technology and the pandemic changed the way we connect or don't connect with each other. If we feel we belong, then we do lots for that group or person.

In a world where loneliness and social isolation is on the rise, the feeling of belonging is even more important. Of course, the opposite is the feeling of exclusion; felt by many who have been hurt by other people's behaviour. As a coping mechanism, many choose to withdraw when left out of general party invitations or experience cliques.

I feel that I belong to my son and my husband, some long-time friends, who are my pretend family and some new friends in the village and to the church. So what are your answers?

If you want to belong then maybe, you need to reach out. Remember you are never alone with a book or a phone.

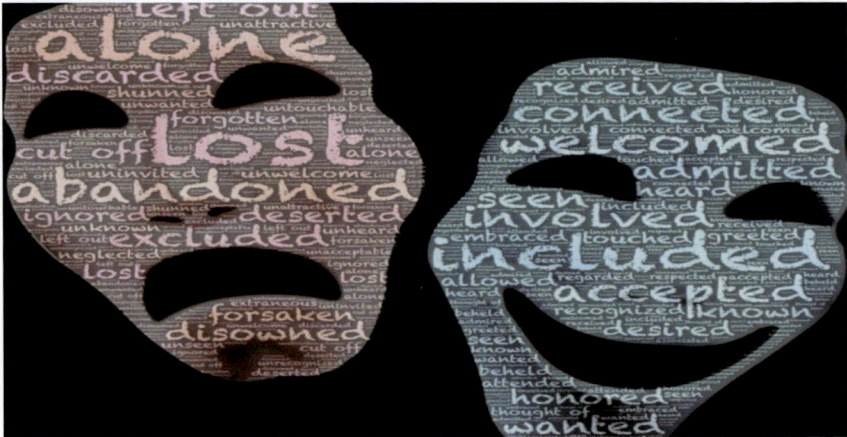

19. Uncertainty

I heard this word 23 times in one day on the media. So yes, uncertainty is everywhere from government to hospital deaths and a lack of the certainty of when it will end and when a vaccine will be found to end the anxiety in so many people's daily schooling, working or retiring lives.

How certain are you of your future plans? Are your thoughts ranging from those you have for Christmas, or your own religious celebration dates, or holidays, to the fear of losing your job. Or not being able to find enough money for your everyday expenses of a home or for enough food to eat or heat your home?

The psychology and mental health of our country is at stake. If you're like most people, uncertainty can cause you tremendous anxiety. Why? Because your survival brain is constantly updating your world, making judgments about what's safe and what isn't. Due to its disdain for uncertainty, it makes up all sorts of untested stories hundreds of times a day because, to the mind, uncertainty equals danger.

If your brain doesn't know what's around the corner, it can't keep you out of harm's way. It always assumes the worst, over-personalises threats, and jumps to conclusions. (Your brain will do almost anything for the sake of certainty.) And you're hardwired to overestimate threats and underestimate your ability to handle them—all in the name of survival. Having an end day in mind helps.

When certainty is questioned, your stress response goes haywire, instantly arousing your stress response, and giving you a feeling of fear whether it be about the safety of your health or that of a loved one. The psyche attempts to spur you into action and to get you to safety.

Waiting for certainty can feel like torture by a million tiny cuts. Sometimes the brain prefers to know an outcome one way or another to take the edge off.

Studies show that you're calmer anticipating pain than anticipating uncertainty because pain is certain. Scientists have found that job uncertainty, for example, takes a greater toll on your health than actually losing the job. Statistics also show you're more likely to maintain the stamina to continue taking risks after a car crash than after a series of psychological setbacks.

British researchers discovered that study participants who knew for sure they would receive a painful electric shock felt calmer and less agitated than those who were told they only had a 50% chance of getting the electric shock. Uncertainty makes it worse.

Simultaneously the brain can think positive things and if you think good thoughts you feel good. Negative thinking brings negativity to your health both physically and mentally. Look at all the benefits of the time you spent in lock down. Yes, there have been some, what were yours?

As I write this I am surrounded by the horror of the news about Ukraine, like most people I would struggle to find any benefits of such an atrocity;

that of wanting power, wealth, state ship, ownership and control.

The issue of uncertainty has never been so painful as it must be for all the people in this present war.

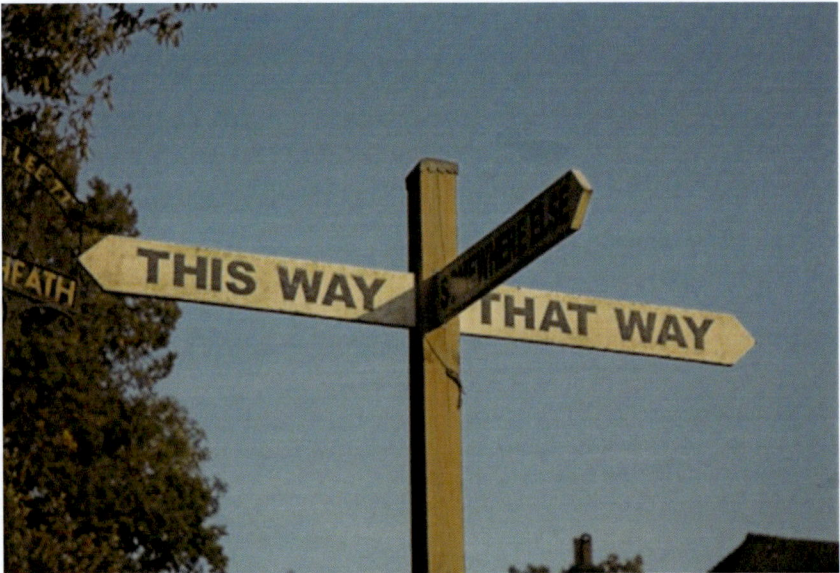

20. Bereavement

Death is the one certain thing that we will all experience. Yet it is still something that so many people find very difficult to talk about. It is swept under the carpet like sex used to be in the early Victorian days. The double standards of the great pomp and circumstance attached to the seen ritual church going practices, whilst the 'Man of the house' would be having illicit sex with his mistresses or servants.

You will most likely have heard the saying 'In the midst of life, we are in death.' It is very difficult to prepare, for even expected deaths.

So how can we handle the loss? We all deal with death in different ways. Like the differing coping mechanisms, we have: Frantic activity, withdrawal, packaging, fight, flight or freeze. Some of us will do frantic activity to avoid thinking or feeling, whilst others want to withdraw. Many emotions are experienced, anger, guilt, emptiness, grief, depression, frustration, sadness, loss and relief. The last one is often when someone has been in a lot of pain beforehand.

There are stages and phases that we go through, though not necessarily in this chronological order. As our moods swing, one day we can feel one thing and the next day something quite different.

These are the phases:

Denial – is a feeling of isolation and disbelief. Some days even forgetting that your loved one has died and maybe buying flowers for them without remembering that they have died.

Anger – irrational anger towards the deceased, then feeling guilt then anger again; *how could they leave me?*

Bargaining – trying to gain control by again asking 'if only' in a bid to change the inevitable.

Depression – feelings are turned inwards and depression is a blanket over inturned anger. Maybe privately wondering how we will cope without them.

We all seem to need 'closure' according to the media and that eventually leads us to 'get over the death' but we don't want closure we need to continue with the grieving links and pathways to and with our loved ones. We need to rejoice in their memory not mourn their loss.

Acceptance – that means that we know and accept that the loved one is dead and will not return. We start to withdraw and find a calmness. Then we can see beyond the death and remember their life as a whole. Sometimes though, we may want to delay our recovery. It is as if the mind is thinking it will mean that I did not love them if I accept their death and continue living and laughing.

Handling bereavement is not just about death, it is also about loss. So often the loss of a parent in a divorce or the separation of a child's parents or the loss of a close friend or lover or a special person in our lives. Loss is not just experienced by children but adults too when relationships break down.

For pet lovers you also know the immense pain of the death of a pet. You could not have loved them more if you had fertilised them or have given birth to them.

Recognise that grieving doesn't have time boundaries, it takes as long as it takes. Try to continue to be available to listen, not just immediately but for as long as it takes.

Think and Feel Acceptance Not Closure

So many times, we hear the media talk about 'now you have closure'. We don't want closure, we want acceptance. Because when someone that we love dies, we want to be able to recall our special memories, which can be triggered by so many incidental things; a comment, music, a book, TV, a play, hearing their name, recalling a part of their life. It is not until we reach an acceptance stage in the grieving process, that we can begin to celebrate our memories.

Writing this just after Easter in an atmosphere of such suffering with so many deaths due to the Coronavirus epidemic, when so many thousands of people will be grieving. There would be no Christians if we had had closure on Good Friday, Christians would not want closure but the acceptance that Christ rose from the dead. Other religions also have acceptance about their faith.

For many of us we are in lockdown with time to think rather than being involved in our usual frantic activity. Our life is made up of time, so waste your time and you waste your life. The psyche is very powerful and you can use it positively or negatively.

We have a feeling brain and a thinking brain, the feeling brain is greater that the thinking brain when we are feeling a lot of emotion, the thinking brain can shut down. Do you believe that how you think affects how you feel? Yes? Then do you believe that how you feel affects how you think? Yes? Then do you believe that how you feel affects how you behave? Yes? So, thinking and feeling positively and being appreciative for what is being done for us, is likely to affect how we behave towards others and towards ourselves.

In these times of so much death whilst we need to give ourselves permission to grieve, we also need to give ourselves permission to be happy in the memory of our loved ones.

We do not want closure we want acceptance to celebrate the love, if we had it, not to continue mourning the loss.

Whichever religion we follow, or whether we are an agnostic or atheist, almost all of us can find comfort in the belief of the everlasting life of our memories.

Loved or hated – people's bodies may die and leave us but our memories will live forever, until we suffer memory loss.

Tears mean that there was Love.

Grief is the price we pay for Love.

Without attachment there would be no grief or sense of loss.

There has been a great deal of media coverage about mental illness with the admissions of many celebrities alongside Princes William and Harry, about their mental anguish of trying to deal with the death of their mother and how to handle their depression.

Death is the one thing that we will all experience. Yet it is still something that many people find very difficult to talk about. It is swept under the carpet, not talked about and certainly not easily or openly discussed, rather like sex in the Victorian early days.

Have you experienced bereavement of a loved one?

How did you manage your grief? Are you grieving right now for someone? Are you still grieving for the death of someone who died years, even decades, ago?

So many people carry their grief throughout their life without ever revealing or resolving their inner feelings about what the death of that person meant to them and how it had affected them.

Death brings out in us so many emotions; anger, guilt, emptiness, grief, depression, frustration, sadness, loss and relief. The last one because often when someone has been in a lot of pain beforehand there is relief in us that their pain is now over.

Death is a very difficult thing for which we can prepare ourselves, even when we have been expecting it for some times. That applies to both ourselves and others. Do use the word died not lost or passed away or other avoidance words it helps you to reach acceptance of the fact.

What happens to us psychologically when we try to handle loss? We all deal with death in different ways. We have differing coping strategies. Some of us will do frantic activity to avoid thinking or feeling about the loss of the person concerned, whilst others of us just want to hide, be alone and withdraw. What do you do when you grieve?

Psychologically there are several stages and phases that we go through, though not necessarily in a chronological order.

As our moods swing, one day we can feel one thing and the next day feel something quite different. It is believed that these stages are;

Denial – a feeling of isolation and disbelief.

Anger – an irrational anger towards the deceased, then feeling guilt then anger again.

Bargaining – we try to gain control again by talking to ourselves and asking 'if only' in a bid to try to change the inevitable. However simultaneously privately wondering how we will cope without them.

Depression – our feelings are turned inwards and depression is a blanket over our inturned anger. We need what is commonly called 'closure' and that eventfully comes with –

Acceptance – we know and accept that the loved one is dead and will not return. We start to withdraw and find a calmness. Then we can see beyond the death and remember their life as a whole. Sometimes though we may want to delay recovery.

The idea of closure is wrong. We never close our memories whether good or bad but we can learn to complete any unfinished business. We can change painful feelings into painful memories. Whether you believe in everlasting life or not you will believe that there is everlasting life in your mind of a loved one. Their influence and memories can be resurrected suddenly maybe by a name, with a particular song or tune, a book, a date, music, film, play or a place.

Bereavement and the emotions involved, is not just about death; it is also for a child, about the loss of a parent in a separation or in the divorce of their parents, as well as the loss of a lover, partner or loving close friend.

For pet lovers you will also know the immense pain of the death of a pet. You could not have loved them more if you had given birth to them.

If you are supporting someone who is trying to handle a death then recognise that grieving doesn't have time boundaries, it takes as long as it takes. Try to continue to be available for them, to listen, not just immediately but for as long as it takes.

People are so kind when it just happens, "Call me anytime day or night I'll be there."

Try ringing after a few weeks, you are expected to be fine now and certainly after a year. Do note the date, the anniversary may not register with you but that date will be imprinted and engraved forever in the mind of the griever.

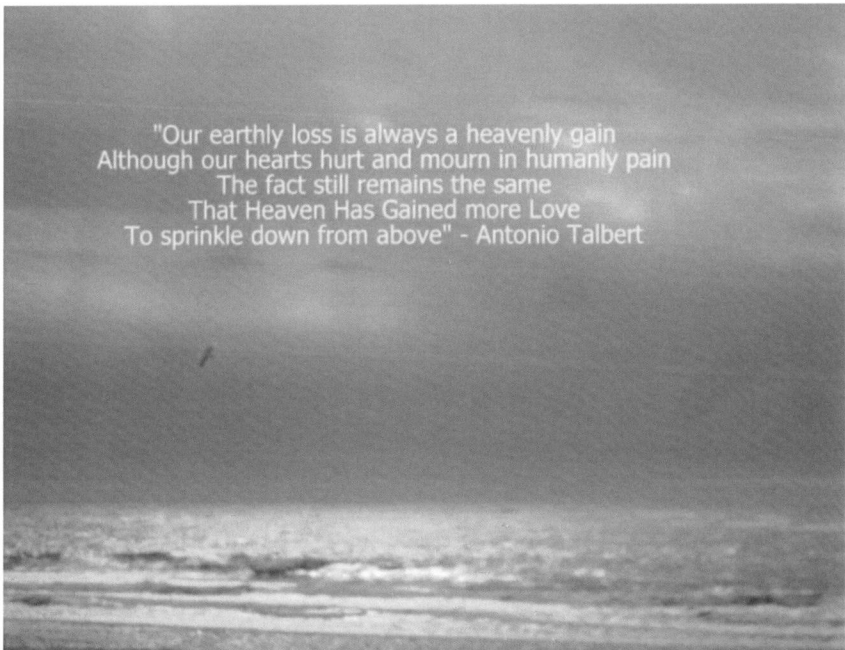

"Our earthly loss is always a heavenly gain
Although our hearts hurt and mourn in humanly pain
The fact still remains the same
That Heaven Has Gained more Love
To sprinkle down from above" - Antonio Talbert

21. Grieving for the Death of a Pet

I don't want to write this. The reason being that our dog Zip died a few days ago and the psychology of grieving for a pet is the same as for a human. They are the same stages as we talked about earlier.

I am in denial, so by writing this I am having to come to terms with accepting that it is true. We rescued Zip when he was 18 months old approximately the RSPA cannot be sure of their age when they find them abandoned in Ireland, or anywhere else. He was around 14 when he died.

He had been beaten, became terrified if accidently you raised your hand with anything in it, like a brush. He would cower, tremble and wee a little. He was a stressed, nervous, hyper anxious, frightened dog. He didn't bark for six months but was the most communicative dog we had ever had. He grunted, playfully pulled at your clothes, made childlike noises of asking to be played with, or walked or fed. Or just to show you that he was happy and wanted to have some fun with you. When he eventually did bark, he scared himself and then wagged his tail furiously wide and fast in delight.

I believe that when we go to a funeral, we go to every other funeral that we have attended. Similarly, when we experience the death of a pet (or a human) we open the psychological floodgates of others that we have loved and lost. So, some of my tears were for my mum.

My mum died when I was seven on her thirty-third birthday, she had been in the hospital for a month, can you believe that in those days you were not allowed to take children to visit people in hospitals but I was given special permission to be allowed to go in just on her birthday. I sent her a card in a box with 1/3p written in pencil on the back and my dad took it in. He came home to tell me that she had died and I asked, "Did she see my card?"

"No, she died before she opened it," he replied.

You don't have to be a psychologist, therapist or anything to know that sometimes the kindest thing to do is to lie to a child in grief. I wanted to hear how she loved it and me for sending it, and it was the best card that she had ever seen.

What helps us to handle the loss? Be prepared to feel the loss; to not sleep or to sleep longer, to not want to eat or to overeat, to get rid of all your pet's things or to have them as a keepsake, to get another pet or to not want another pet ever. There is no right or wrong way to grieve, do whatever you want to when you are ready.

However, some people say 'it was only a dog', keep away from them. Talk to those who empathise with you. One good thing is that we have no 'unfinished business' with pets. You do not regret what you said or what they said, or dwell on their failure to be a faithful partner, or remember their times of betrayal or losing trust, anger or even violence.

Grief feels terrible. It is also a sign that you shared a deep, sacred love with your pet. I bet you wouldn't trade your grief for any of those wonderful, loving, fun times you shared with your pet! Unfortunately, grief is the price we pay for loving deeply. Thank you, friends, for your love and thank you Zip.

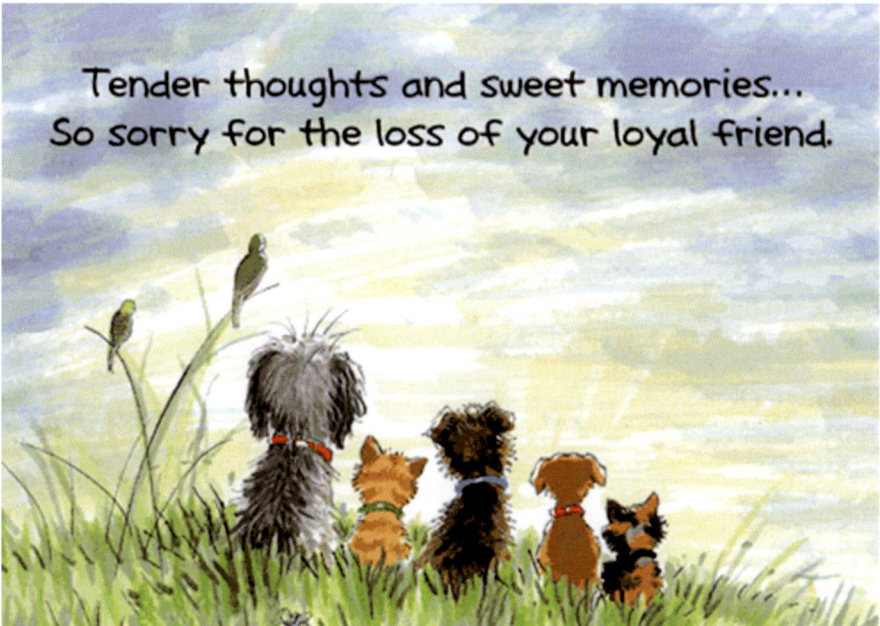

Tender thoughts and sweet memories...
So sorry for the loss of your loyal friend.

22. The Power of Touch

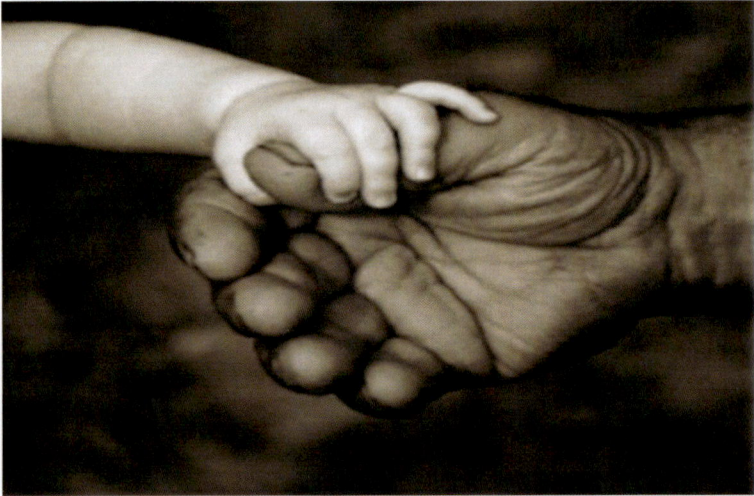

Touch is the first sense we acquire and the secret weapon in many a successful relationship. Likely to lead to mental wellness.

Many psychological studies have been tested as to how touch influences us in our attitude to others. In one case librarians – people returning books were asked how helpful the two staff were. The one that was instructed to touch their hand was perceived as the more helpful one. Waitresses and waiters are found to be given larger tips if they touch the customer appropriately at some point.

I was so sad to hear on the news, that foster parents were being warned to not touch or cuddle their foster children and that foster dads should avoid being alone in a car with their foster child, on school runs.

What nonsense – you are either a loving foster parent or you should not be in that paid position and role, if your behaviour towards children is suspected.

When we touch someone their oxytocin levels go up, heart rates go down, all these wonderful things happen that you can't see. You can't touch without being touched. A lot of those same beneficial psychological and physiological consequences happen to the person touching.

Research has revealed that a person giving a massage or a hug, experiences as great a reduction in stress hormones as the person on the receiving end.

The number of paedophiles in this country are point naught, naught one percent and yet the rest of the teaching fraternity are prevented from touching children when they are upset, distressed or even physically hurt. In Scotland nursery schools were advised a decade ago that you should not put a three-year-old child on your knee if s/he was crying.

What prompts such statements and from whom, again, that irrational fear that everybody is about to abuse young children?

Children most certainly do need to be protected from preying adults (as aid charities should know). According to the experts on child protection it is fine to touch children's shoulders or upper arms.

As well as children, adults also need warmth and touch. How many male parents and grandparents do you know, who are now anxious about cuddling, playing physical contact games, bathing their children or grandchildren, taking a lost child by the hand – in case they are seen as a paedophile?

Both children and adults know when you are touching them for support and with love! Whatever happened to the knowledge that you can say so much more with a touch, it can mean so much more than speaking with a thousand words?

It is so sad that many senior citizens homes and flats do not allow pets for the touch of a pet and fondling them brings all of us to a mentally healthy place.

Behaviour

23. Why Do Humans Resist Change?

Do you like change? Changing your house, your interior design, your garden, your habits, your clothes, your friends, your food, your hobbies, your car, your religious or political beliefs, your holidays or your values? I do. Friends know me well, are aware that I am always moving furniture, garden tubs and I have lived in 31 different houses,

> Change can be scary, but you know what's scarier? Allowing Fear to stop you from Growing, Evolving, and Progressing.
> -mandy hale-
> WWW.LIVELIFEHAPPY.COM

bought 20 of them. What a wonderful opportunity for a fresh start and new experiences.

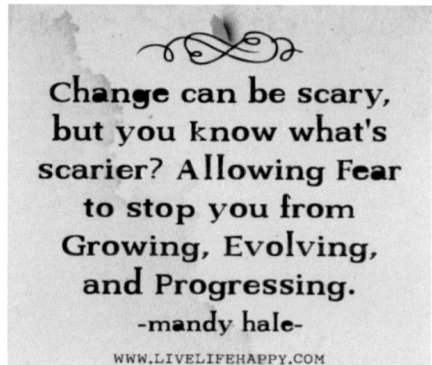

Whilst many of us may welcome change still many others may resist it. Why do humans resist change? It is because of a fear of the loss of control. Change interferes with autonomy and can make people feel that they've lost control over their territory. It's not just political, as in who has the power. Our sense of self-determination is often the first thing to go when we are faced with a potential change coming from someone else.

When you and I try to convince someone to change, we call it **persuasion.** However, when someone tries to get us to do something that we don't want to do, we call it **nagging and confrontational**. Our double-standard is based on whether we are giving or receiving the suggested change. Or when we think that we know, or think we know better. It won't work, even without trying the change. We tend to use double standards when either we care a lot; or when we are short of alternatives.

Based on rigorous research, individuals move through five stages of behavioural change; **precontemplation** (imagining it); **contemplation** (wondering about the implication), **preparation** (getting ready), **action** (doing it), and **maintenance** (keeping up the change or not).

That means the adoption of healthy behaviours or the cessation of unhealthy ones. People may oscillate back and forth between the various steps for many months or years before achieving long-lasting change in their healthy behaviour.

The fear of change or changing things is called **metathesiophobia.** It is often linked with **tropophobia** which is the fear of moving. The origin of the word metathesiophobia comes from Greek 'meta' meaning change and phobos meaning fear.

You can never cross the ocean until you have the courage to lose sight of the shore (Christopher Columbus, 1492)

24. Racism

"I am a racist."

This is how Sheila Hancock started her talk about her new book, several years ago when I attended a national book day conference, in London of celebrity authors, chaired by Sandy Toxig.

Sheila went on to explain, that she was talking about the Germans. As an elderly woman growing up in the Second World War, she was conditioned to hate the Germans. She went on to say how many Germans were now her friends whom she loved and respected, once she had got to know them as individuals and had spent time in their country.

Babies are not born racists. We acquire our first attitudes from the significant people in our early lives and from then on, our experiences of living, working and socialising with people from different races. Where we live, the people whom we meet, our education, our work, the type of careers we follow, the partners that we choose, our families, our friends, our religion or not, the goals which we pursue and our values will undoubtedly also influence us.

As a young child in my first Sunday school, I was given a text card with a picture of Jesus surrounded by children of every nationality with the words "suffer little children to come unto me".

I kept this for many years and it initiated my strong belief that everybody is born equal. I have heard many people say 'rubbish of course we are not born equal.' Of course, we are not, not in terms of money, having a loving family, or even a family, being loved, being physically and mentally healthy, having access to education or to medical care, or of equal intelligence or having equal opportunities. But we are born equal in terms of our feelings... Almost everybody wants to feel loved, valued, wanted, respected, kindness, worthy and that they matter.

Not judged by the colour of their skin, their physical or mental health, their poverty, addictions, lack of a particular cultural background, their sexuality, age, religion, their dwelling, their money – but seen as someone, whoever they are, as an emotional human being who may feel hurt and rejected by our behaviour towards them.

I was brave enough when I was 17 years old and training as an NNEB student working in a day nursery alternate week in inner Manchester, to report to our head of the nursery nursing training college how racist the matron was. She had said of one of the black families 'they're all right when they are little with their plaits and red bows, but it's when they grow up you can see how we think that they came from monkeys'. As part of my training we had to write a thesis (long essay) of our choosing, I chose to write about 'Colour Bar in Britain' it was three month's work and for me it was a very emotional piece of writing. The teacher's simple, one comment at the end was 'There is no colour bar in Britain.'

What do I know about what the black and ethnic minorities feel in Britain? As I now live in a La La Land white village, with less than one percent black community, few children, a significantly large number of retired residents and many gay residents.

I think a lot of people, outwardly pleasant, do hold internalised racist views. Do you? What I do know is that I am not a racist and as a young child was anti-racism.

Are you?

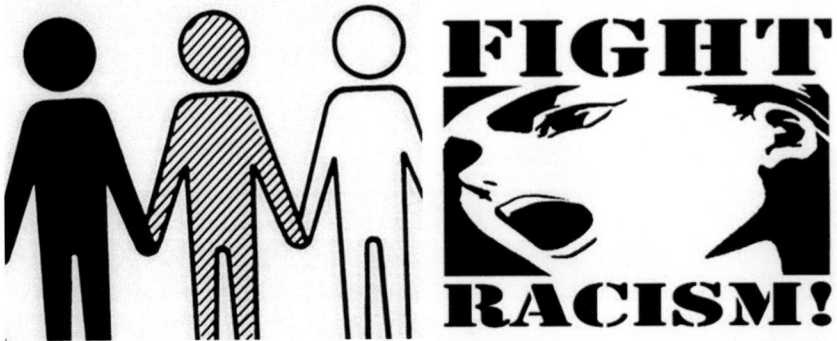

25. Bullying

What Is Bullying?

Bullying is an attempt to frighten or intimidate someone. It can take many different forms and can mean being teased, criticised, ignored or left out, being called names, told that you are stupid or having rumours spread about you.

Bullying can mean receiving intimidating notes or unpleasant telephone messages. It can be physical; being pushed, pawed, hit or even attacked. Bullying can mean being forced to hand over money or possessions or being forced to do something that is illegal.

The bully may try to single you out and exclude you from the group, denying you friendship, information or support – this is called victimisation, targeting or mobbing.

Bullying at work can mean taking credit for another person's work or trying to over-rule someone's authority. It can be setting impossibly high targets, not delegating, withholding information or removing responsibility. The bully may refuse reasonable requests, interfere with post or other types of communication and use lengthy memos or emails to make wild or inaccurate accusations.

Bullying Is...

- Being teased
- Being called names
- Receiving offensive emails or mobile messages
- Being ignored and left out
- Having rumours spread about you
- Being denied information
- Being denied support
- Being denied friendship

- Being pushed or pawed
- Being hit or attacked
- Being embarrassed
- Being humiliated
- Being forced to hand over money or possessions.
- Being made to do something that is illegal

Management or Bullying?

A few managers believe that they can only manage by bullying. They abuse their position by humiliating and belittling staff, rather than concentrating on motivating them. Bullying management can become part of the organisational culture and organisations of this type generally have high levels of absenteeism and staff turnover.

Overt bullying is relatively easy to recognise but bullying may consist of constant critical verbal and written communications – in particular emails or memos copied to a number of people – undermining the confidence of employees.

Why Do People Bully Others?

Bullies are usually people who feel insecure, sometimes because someone is bullying them, or they were bullied as children. A manager who bullies may be being bullied himself or herself, by someone above them.

A child who was constantly criticised or humiliated, or never allowed to show their feelings may develop into a bully. Aggressive relationships may be all they have ever experienced. Some people believe that certain personality types are prone to bullying behaviour.

Bullies are usually disliked because their behaviour towards others is threatening. They may find it difficult to have normal open, friendly relationships. Because they are insecure, bullies particularly dislike people who are popular, clever, friendly and successful.

Bullies are often good liars – especially when challenged about their behaviour – and they are often charming in the presence of others. They hide behind a mask of innocence that conceal their insecurity and deceit. They may have low self-esteem.

Who Do They Bully?

- **Popular people**: especially those who are liked by their colleagues
- **Successful people**: especially those who are good at the things in which the bully would like to succeed
- **Vulnerable people:** especially if they are going through family problems
- **Minority groups**: especially if they belong to a different race or culture
- **People with a different religion from themselves:** because the bully may lack empathy and understanding
- **People with mental disabilities**: makes the bullies feel superior
- **People with physical disabilities**: make the bully feel physically superior

What Can You Do If You Are Being Bullied?

Remember that the bully has the problem, not you! It isn't your fault that this is happening. Believe in yourself.

Don't suffer in silence, share your problem with someone else. Try talking to a friend, colleague or anyone that you trust and let them help you to keep things in perspective. Maybe the bully doesn't realise that their behaviour is hurting you.

People often feel that management won't do anything about bullying, but it is your right to tell a line manager that you are being bullied and transfer some of the burden onto their shoulders. You don't have to let that person take over. You can talk with them about what you would like to happen.

Remember sharing your problem will help, but suffering alone will ultimately lead to depression and stress.

Try not to give up, it *is* possible to learn to cope and learning to be more assertive is important. If you *act* in an assertive way you will *feel* more in control.

Being assertive is quite different from being aggressive. An assertive person stands upright and looks people in the eye, speaks clearly and starts a sentence with the word 'I' and not 'you'.

"I don't like you speaking to me in that way ..."

Practising what you want to say in advance and paying attention to your body language will make you feel more confident.

A passive person lowers their eyes, clasps their hands and shows everyone that they feel inadequate and insecure, these are 'victim' signals.

What Can You Do If Someone Else Is Being Bullied?

Bullying usually affects a number of people. If you witness anyone being bullied, make it clear that you don't approve of the behaviour, discuss it with others and if you feel it is necessary, report it.

Bullies try to isolate their victims; you can help by being aware of this and helping to prevent it.

What Can the Organisation Do?

A responsible organisation needs an anti-bullying policy. Involving staff representatives in the creation of a policy will raise awareness of the issues involved – staff will become more aware of their own behaviour and its effect on others.

Some people don't realise that their behaviour is viewed by others as bullying and a company-wide discussion of the issues can help all staff to understand the problem.

What Should the Policy Include?

- What is meant by bullying and harassment?
- How incidents of bullying will be dealt with?
- How to complain and who to complain to?
- Staff training in assertiveness skills, managing stress, avoiding conflict and everyday counselling

The Organisational Costs of Bullying

- Absenteeism
- Lost time
- Stress
- Costs of new recruiting and retraining
- Tribunal proceedings

- Loss of public image
- Loss of profits

The Hidden Costs Are –

The emotional energy that is used in dealing with the psychological upset to all colleagues affected by bullying.

What Can Good Managers Do?

- Have an anti-bullying policy and follow it
- Set a good example
- Be an honest, open, genuine role model to your staff
- Treat staff as emotional human beings
- Respect and value them
- Speak to staff, rather than communicating through emails and memos
- Remember that staff grow with praise and shrivel with criticism

Deal with bullying promptly

- Act against unreasonable behaviour
- Comment on offensive attitudes
- Let staff know how to report bullying incidents
- Deal with complaints now and do not turn 'a blind eye'
- Nip conflict 'in the bud' to avoid it escalating to disciplinary procedures
- Establish a 'no blame' culture at work

Fact: In 84% of UNISON case studies – bullies have bullied before, although management knew all about it, only one in four managers did anything about it.

Handling Bullying Complaints

It is important to listen to both people involved and to recognise that they need help. Spend time with each of them so that they can talk at length about the underlying issues. Confidentiality is essential.

Explain what bullying is, but condemn the *behaviour* and not the person. Realise that there are almost always two sides to a story and that in many cases there is equal blame.

After you have heard the story, ask permission to deal with the issue. Take the matter seriously, be sympathetic and empathetic. Offer choices like 'ignore' or 'address the incident'.

Try to understand how both the victim and the bully are feeling. Let the bully know how the other person is feeling. Realise that it is often a difference of perceptions. Ask the bully what sort of behaviour they perceive as bullying.

You may be able to ask the two people involved to face each other and to say what happened (their version), how they feel and what they need.

Respond to the people involved quickly and without delay.

Bullying in Schools

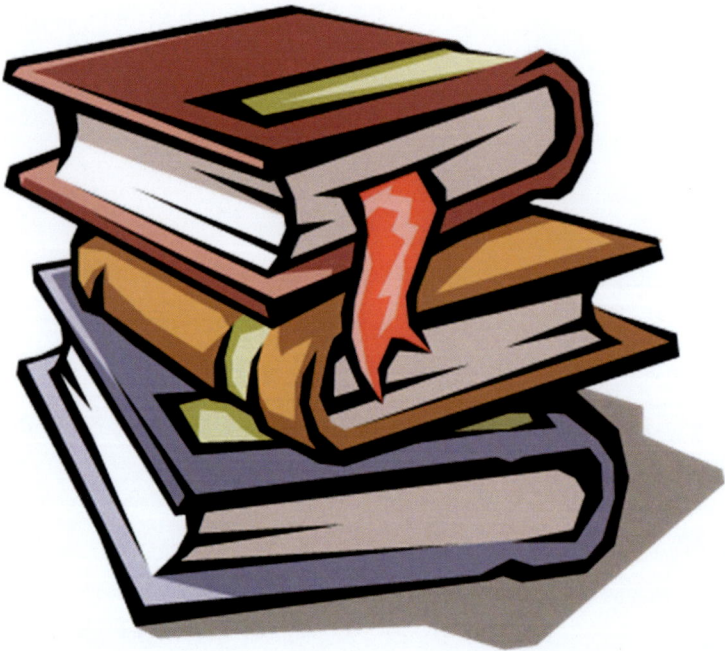

What Is Bullying?

Bullying can mean many different things

- Being attacked because of your physical appearance, religion or race
- Being called names
- Being forced to hand over money or possessions.
- Being hit or attacked
- Being ignored and left out

Being made to do something that is illegal

- Being pushed or pawed
- Being teased
- Having rumours spread about you
- Having your bag or other possessions taken and thrown away
- Told that you are stupid

So Bullying is being

- Ignored and side-lined
- Belittled
- Constantly criticised
- Denied friendship
- Denied information
- Denied support
- Embarrassed
- Encouraged to feel guilty
- Group bullying (being excluded)
- Humiliated
- Name-calling
- Not being spoken to
- Receiving intimidating notes
- Receiving unpleasant telephone messages
- Singled out

- Threatened

Hence Bullying Behaviour Can Be

- Abusive
- Aggressive
- Behaving like their parent or role model
- Devious and sly
- Forceful
- Hostile
- Humiliating
- Insensitive
- Intimidating
- Lying
- Oppressive
- Threatening
- Using offensive language

What Do Bullies Do?

- Call you names
- Write hateful things about you
- Send offensive mobile memos
- Leave you out of the group
- Don't talk to you
- Threaten you
- Scare you
- Make sexual comments about you
- Use sarcasm
- Cut across your conversations
- Spread malicious rumours about you
- Ridicule
- Hit or punch you
- Tell you to do things you don't want to

Because they are insecure, bullies do not like people who are

- Competent
- Creative
- Genuine
- Helpful
- Honest
- Imaginative
- Incorruptible
- Innovative
- Liked (by friends or teachers)
- Popular
- Sensitive
- Slow to anger
- Successful
- Trustworthy

So they select:

Popular people
Especially those who are liked by their teachers and have friends.

Successful people
Especially those who are good at the things in which they would like to succeed.

Vulnerable people
Especially if they are going through family problems.

Minority groups
Especially if they belong to a different race or culture.

People with a different religion from themselves
Because they are often ignorant and lack empathy.

People with mental disabilities

Because usually they are not too bright themselves, so they can feel superior.

People with physical disabilities

Because they are often cowards, they temporarily feel brave.

So, bullies are often

Liars, when their bullying is addressed.

Charming, in the presence of others.

Hiding, behind an innocent mask to conceal their insecurity and deceit.

Remember adults can also be bullies.

Mums, dads, sisters, brothers, grandparents, stepparents, parent's partners, teachers –

They are all capable of making you feel bad about yourself.

So find an adult to whom you can talk. There are lots of caring sensitive adults about, honestly.

Adults can also bully each other.

Can you think of a teacher who bullies another teacher, or an adult who bullies another adult?

Some reasons why bullies bully!

- 'A cruel streak in them'
- A bullying role model
- Amoral
- Are insecure
- Are unable to express emotions and feelings
- Being bullied
- Constantly criticised as a child
- Control
- Cowardly
- Different values
- Experienced aggressive relationships
- Fear
- Feel threatened

- Feel unloved, not valued
- Given negative messages about themselves at home or at school
- Greed
- Have been bullied
- Ignorance
- Jealousy
- Just 'year eight' boys
- Lack a sense of belonging
- Lack interpersonal skills to form clean, open honest relationships
- Living up to expectations of teacher's family, peers
- Lucrative
- Nastiness
- Not allowed to show their feelings so unable to verbally express their emotions
- Peer pressure
- Power
- They don't know how to deal with their anger
- They feel inadequate
- They have been criticised or humiliated as a child
- They have family problems
- To be popular
- To gain attention
- To temporarily feel good about themselves

All this means a lack of self-love so low self esteem
What can you do?

- Ask your parents to visit the school.
- Be assertive.
- Don't give up.

Ignore them

It is your right to tell an adult that you are being bullied and transfer some of the burden on to their shoulders. You don't have to let them takeover. You can talk with them about what you would like to happen.

Keep things in perspective.

Practice what you want to say
Remember that emotions govern behaviour.

Remember that prejudice is built on fear and ignorance and remember that teachers have to listen carefully when a child tells them about being bullied.

Remember that they have the problem, not you!
Talk it over what you can do with a friend, teacher, your mum or dad or anyone that you trust.

Tell an adult that you can trust
Tell someone.
Use your humour.

Violence is built on frustration
'What you think is what you feel,' so think positively.

What Can You Do in Schools?

Write down what happened.

What Can Parents Do About It?

Try to empower your child to tell their teacher.

If they cannot then you tell the head teacher or their teacher.

Human nature being what it is, most teachers are more likely to do something about it if their head teacher has been informed.

Most schools will have a pastoral care system so try to talk to their personal tutors.

Most of these staff are trained to be empathic and tend to have caring values rather than considering that it is yet another intrusion on their time.

As a parent do not encourage more violence with violence. If your son or daughter does respond in the same way as the bully, then often they are the one to be seen and are reprimanded and named as the bully.

- Name-calling and teasing
- Take a holistic approach
- See both individually to ascertain both sides of the story then bring them together
- Highlight the effect that the behaviour is having on the other person
- Actively listen, that is with ears, eyes, brain and heart
- Listen to all the views surrounding the incident
- Ask yourself 'is this an accurate account of events?'
- Realise that it is often a difference of perceptions
- Find out the reason and cause
- Confidentiality is essential
- Establish confidentiality within legal limits
- After the story ask permission to deal with the issue
- Raise awareness
- Talk it over
- Offer choices like 'ignore', 'respond in similar way' or 'address the incident'
- Point out that we all have choices but each choice has a consequence
- Get back quickly to the people involved
- Establish a 'no blame' culture
- Take the matter seriously
- Be sympathetic and empathetic
- Use peer group counselling

How Can Significant Adults Help?

Listen to both people involved.

Recognise that they need help.

Spend time with them so that they can talk at length about the underlying issues.

Try to understand how both the victim and the bully are feeling.

Let the bully know how the other person is feeling.

Ask the bully what sort of behaviour they perceive as bullying.

Define bullying to them.

Condemn the behaviour – not the person.

Realise that there are almost always two sides to most stories and that in many cases there is often a situation by where there is equal blame.

The response may have been because of the stimulus. Someone may unexpectedly resort to bullying.

'You're a mummy's boy' could greatly hurt, if the child's father has left the family home and he loves both of them but is torn between bitter, combative parents.

Try to get them to face each other and to say what happened (in their truth), how they feel and what they need.

What Can Be Done About It, In Schools, To Stop It?

Teachers and pupils can set an example, by treating people as emotional human beings.

- Be consistent in your approach to bullying behaviour.
- Have a working policy, in school, which pupils understand.
- Try to deal with it efficiently and effectively.
- Use sanctions.
- Peer coercion.
- Involve parents.
- Have awareness raising lessons.
- Consider self-defence instruction.
- Set up peer counselling training groups.

Teach

- Assertiveness skills.
- Interpersonal skills.
- Early childhood scripting and how it later affects the adult.
- About group bullying, and the effect of exclusion.
- Role-play alternative ways of dealing with bullying.
- Facilitate change of role of bully and bullied to see the others viewpoint.
- In a student-centred way and ask pupils what they see or experience as bullying.
- How to address conflict.

- How to deal with criticism effectively.

What Can You Do?

Report it.

When, who and where giving details of the bullying incident and any witnesses.

What Stops Children from Reporting It?

They suffer in silence because of fear of:

- Teachers won't do anything about it
- Future abuse
- Loss of friends
- Depression
- Stress

What Can Heads and Teachers Do?

Treat People as Emotional Human Beings.

- Respect and value them
- Act on unreasonable behaviour
- Comment on offensive attitudes
- Let staff know how to report bullying incidents
- Deal with complaints now
- Do not turn 'a blind eye'

Be an honest, open, genuine role model to your staff.

Nip conflict' in the bud' to avoid it escalating to disciplinary procedures.

Speak to staff, rather than constantly communicating through emails and memos.

Remember that almost everybody grows with praise and shrivels with criticism. Adults and children alike

Exclusion – should only be as a last resort!

To assist anyone that is being bullied use the 'empty chair 'method of counselling.

Let the person talk out loud to an empty chair, imagining that the bully is there and say what they would really like to say. Then change places and become the bully, responding to what the 'bullied person' has just been saying.

Support Staff Training That Involves

- Assertiveness skills
- Awareness of the effects of unacceptable behaviour
- Effective interpersonal and intrapersonal skills
- Emotional intelligence
- Empathising with differing values, cultures, sexuality and disability
- Every day counselling skills
- How to change attitudes
- How to complain
- How to identify bullying
- Managing stress
- Policies for eradicating bullying
- Practical appraisal and interviewing skills
- Skills in handling conflict
- The important use and effect of language

Cost of Getting It Wrong

- Absenteeism
- Time loss
- Stress
- Costs of new recruiting and retraining
- Tribunal proceedings
- Loss of public image

The Hidden Costs Are –

80% of your psychic energy can be lost dealing with the psychological upset to all colleagues affected.

The Law

There is lots of legislation for racial (RRA 1976) and sexual harassment (SDA 1977) however there is very little protection for employees against bullying. You can only rely on unsatisfactory provision of the 1974 Health and Safety Act. Where bullying employees can be penalised for not taking steps to prevent bullying at work as in breach of the implied contractual duty of mutual trust and confidence.

Personal Psychic Profiles – Mind Matters

Now you have the opportunity to see how your mind may affect you with the personal psychic profiles. Your mind matters.

I FIND THAT I CAN BE ASSERTIVE WITH SOME PEOPLE BUT NOT WITH OTHERS, ESPECIALLY WHEN I AM BEING CRITICISED, WHY?

Regardless of how senior or junior, your position is at work, you will have to manage yourself in order to assertively work with others.

Let us begin by highlighting your relationships with people at work. Forget for a moment what you have to manage and concentrate on whom you have to manage or on who manages you. You only have so much energy and time and it is likely that you are spending an inordinate, disproportional amount of time on some staff rather than on others. Your psychic energy level (that is, the amount of energy you use on psychological thinking or worrying about things) is lowered.

You are highly likely to work or play with a mixture of people, some you like, some you don't, some of whom get on with the job, take up little of your time, to whom you can responsibly delegate and who appear to be successfully achieving their targets.

Whilst others seem to always want to talk to you about inconsequential minute details, fall behind on deadlines, lack drive or sparkle and seem to be take up so much of your precious time. It is likely that you will always have such a mixture, but with astute assertive skills you can help some of the people from the latter group into the former one.

Regardless of these two categories, there is probably something more fundamental going on in you. Something, which you may be reluctant to discuss with others. Thoughts, feelings, emotions and attitudes that you hold towards individuals in both groups.

So, let us explore what it is about you and others that can lead to your being non-assertive that is either appeasing or aggressive, with some people, whilst having the skills and the ability to be assertive and effectively work with others.

Therefore, the first stage is to try to identify what is happening for you emotionally. How you are feeling about the people with whom you work. Whether they are people you manage or those who manage you. Then the next stage will be to identify what it is about you that may be creating some of the difficulties that you are encountering.

It probably comes down to very basic needs that you have. Maybe you need to be liked, be right, be quick, be strong, or be seen to be in charge and always trying harder. Whatever drives you will have a knock-on effect on those that you manage.

Perhaps you work with some staff, both senior and junior to yourself, whom you think have been promoted beyond their ability. Whilst there are likely to be other people with whom you work where you feel positive, enjoy their company, think that they are a "good laugh", even possibly feel sexually attracted towards them or intellectually stimulated by them.

Establishing your values

EMOTIONS – WITH WHOM??
Please answer the following questions as honestly as you can.
There are no right or wrong answers.

1. Who do you like at work?   _____
(If you are resistant to the word "like" change it to "get on with" or "enjoy working with" or "with whom do you find is easy to work?")

2. Who do you dislike at work?   _____
(Again, if you are querying the word "dislike", change it into your own preferred language.)

3. Who do you trust at work?   _____
(That is you believe that they will not abuse you to others or relay confidential disclosures).

4. Who have you trusted in the past and now find that this trust has been broken or betrayed? _____
(Found that the person you trusted has now broken that trust. If you cannot think of someone at work, what about outside work?)

5. Who do you think has been promoted beyond their ability?

_____

(Even though they may have the 'qualifications'!)

6. Who intellectually stimulates you? _____
(Think of someone with whom you can pitch your wits against, or enjoy stimulating banter, feeling as though your brain is being stretched.)

7. Who has a good sense of humour? _____
(Think of someone who makes you laugh or have an infectious kind of humour. Maybe they are bubbly and have the ability to uplift people with their persona.)

8. Who do you find sexually attractive? _____

9. To whom do you have positive feelings? _____
(or comments like, "I feel I've known you for years…" "We just seemed to get on so well right from our first introduction or meeting…")

10. To whom do you have negative feelings? _____
(Those phrases like, "There's something about him…" "I don't know what it is about her, but…"; "I can't put my finger on it, but we just don't gel…")

Self Confidence

In order to be assertive you need to be able to speak and act in an open, honest and direct way. You need to be able to contribute to meetings, deal with conflict and express your values and opinions. This requires self- confidence. Assessments 1-3 focus on self- confidence. They try to help you recognize and understand how you think and feel about situations and people, and the impact this has on your behaviour. If you feel confident in yourself your behaviour will naturally be more assertive. If you lack confidence, however, you may behave less assertively.

ASSESSMENT : ANCESTRAL VOICES

Your natural self-confidence can be affected by a number of factors – who is present, their relationship to you and, most significantly, your early childhood messages; how you were told to think, feel or behave when you were small. Although other people may also have affected your self-image – partners, associates or colleagues – these 'ancestral voices' stay with you, 'chatting' to you incessantly, like little creatures sitting on your shoulder. Unless you become aware of them these voices can seriously dent your self-confidence and encourage non-assertive behaviour.

Answer the questions overleaf to discover your ancestral voices. Tick the Yes or the No box for each question. If you are wavering then your answer is probably Yes. Commit yourself; don't leave a question unanswered.

Personal Psychic Profile
Mind matters

[1]

Giving And Receiving Compliments.

To accept a compliment assertively all you really need to say is "Thank you".

Assertiveness is about having the ability to respect and admit your own self-worth, and that of other people. It is not about behaving in appeasing or aggressive manner, yet it is often confused with these responses.

So, how did you do in the Fitness Assessment? Look back to page and make a note of the options you ticked below.

Question 1

Question 2

Question 3

However, how did you respond in your check up?

QUESTION 1

The assertive response is B, "Thank you. That feels good". This response reflects a healthy level of self-confidence   → 5 POINTS

The Appeasing response is A, "Thanks, but I don't really think it's that good". This kind of passive response is putting yourself down and also inadvertently saying to the other person that they are not a very good judge of quality. In fact you are discounting their compliment. It also reflects unhealthy levels of self-esteem, self-worth and self-confidence.   → 0 POINTS

The aggressive response is C, "What are you after?" The type of response is suspicious, attacking and hostile. → 0 POINTS

SCORE

QUESTION 2

For question 2, the assertive response is C. "Well done, first-rate presentation. I really think it went down well with the client". This is recognizing the worth of your colleague and celebrating it. You are giving him or her well-deserved praise without undermining your own worth. → 5 POINTS

The aggressive response is A, "Keep your hands off. This one's mine". This is demonstrating your defensiveness, possessiveness and jealousy, which are all aggressive attributes. → 0 POINTS

The appeasing response was, "Oh well, they'll probably want David, not me, to handle their account from now on". This is really putting yourself down and you are in danger of evoking the self-fulfilling prophesy of failing in the relationship. It reflects unhealthy levels of self-worth and confidence.
→ 0 POINTS

SCORE

QUESTION 3

For question 3, the assertive response is A, "Thanks, I'm absolutely thrilled with the promotion". This response shows that you are able to recognize your achievements without denial or embarrassment. Well done, you have a healthy level of self-worth. → 5 POINTS

The aggressive response is B, "I should think so too, after all the hard work and time that I have put into this company". This is a resentful reaction to someone, demonstrating an angry and antagonistic attitude. → 0 POINTS

The appeasing response is C, "It's a fluke, I don't deserve it" This response shows an inability to believe in your own talent, intelligence, ability and achievement. Again, unhealthy levels of self-worth.   → 0 POINTS

SCORE

Personal Psychic Profile
Mind matters
2

Now to look at the messages that your body may be giving to other people, without your knowing.

POSSIBLE FEELINGS OR THOUGHTS EXHIBITED WITH BODY GESTURES

BODY TALK   **NEGATIVE IMPRESSION TRANSMITTED**

Folded arms	I'm uncomfortable, I don't want to be here'
Crossed legs Turned-up toe'	'Keep your distance' I am uncomfortable with what you are saying or what is being asked of me!
Arms above the head	'One day you'll be as Intelligent as I am'
OR	'I'm much too relaxed to be taking this interview seriously'
Hands above shoulders	De-powering myself

Face – Fingers over lips,	Censoring or lacking or near the mouth confidence about what is being said?
Twirling hair	Anxious, childish, nervous. Some think it is sexy
Pointed finger	Accusative, critical
Twitching leg, heel tapping or finger tapping	Stressed

Hence, it is important to give positive rather than negative messages to people, if you want to be perceived as being assertive.

Some people may find these concepts difficult and respond with " I'm not affected by body language. I don't stereotype people". Well, great, but I believe that you will be affected subconsciously, if not consciously, by how people use their bodies.

Remember, in most communications the breakdown is: content 7%, voice 38%, and body language 55%. This is why paying attention to what you do rather than what you say can be so effective in looking assertive.

Thirteen times more information is available in your non-verbal communication than in your words. Hence try to create rapport. Smile initially; as there is nothing better than your looking relaxed, in order to relax the other person. So how do we relax other people and demonstrate "accepting" body language? Now turn to P 2 to find the prescription for assertive body talk.

Section score-strengths and weaknesses round up
Self-confidence (inner fitness)

What do you now think or feel, that you can do about these issues?
How confident are you about the following? Very or not really

1. Trying to behave in an assertive way
2. Presenting yourself in terms of your body language;
3. Believing that you have psychological 'rights';
4. Accepting compliments;
5. Managing conflict and criticisms;

6. Speaking in Meetings;
7. Recognising your drivers and being able to change the way in which you need to think;
8. Showing your feelings;
9. Saying 'no' to people when you do not want to do what is being asked of you;
10. Using different language in order to express your values and needs more assertively?

Score – give yourself 3 marks for responding 'very' and 1 mark for responding 'not really'.

Total score _____

The higher your score the more confident you are.

Personal Psychic Profile
Mind matters
3

Being Assertive at Meetings

Being in a pack can bring about our ancestral inherent behaviour of flight, fright, freeze or fight. When people are stressed or threatened they feel confused, disorientated and can go into a condition or response known as démodé. This means that, they return to their primeval beginnings and think, "Will it eat me, or will I eat it?"

This may sound extreme for a weekly work meeting, but stop and think about it.

If you answered 'yes' to any of the following questions then;

Your fitness profile would tend to mean;

1. An angry outburst at a meeting?   Fight

2. Someone fearful of losing his or her job?   Fear

3. Someone stressed and leaving or running away from a   Flight
meeting?

4. Someone unable to speak at a meeting?   Freeze

5. Someone being verbally destroyed, humiliated, or patronised?   Freeze

There can also be positive feelings from:

6. Spontaneous laughter?   Fun

7. Mutual support of members.   Friendship

8. An intimacy and rapport.   Fondness

9. Public praise being given.   Fuzzy (Warm)

10. Recognition for status or achievement.   Fame

Personal Psychic Profile
Mind matters
4

Saying 'No'

TO WHOM DO YOU FIND IT DIFFICULT TO SAY 'NO'?
List the people to whom you find it difficult to say 'No':

_____

_____

_____

_____

_____

_____

Now work down your list and ask yourself the following questions.
Write down your answers.

What stops you from saying 'No'?

_____

Do they have anything in common?

_____

Do you empower them?

_____

Are you searching for their approval?

_____

What other reasons?

_____

Personal Psychic Profile

Mind matters

5

Dealing with Manipulation

HOOKS AND DRIVERS

To discover your profile, now complete the following five columns, putting your score next to the question numbers below.

E.g. for column A question 3, if you have answered Yes to question 3 then give yourself 1 mark. If you have a No answer then put a zero.

COLUMN A	COLUMN B	COLUMN C	COLUMN D	COLUMN E
3	4	5	1	6
7	8	10	2	9
14	11	15	13	17
16	12	20	19	18
21	24	22	23	25
---	---	---	---	---
---	---	---	---	---

Now add up your score for all of the separate columns. You will find separate scores for columns ABCD and E.

Where you have a score of 3 or more in one column it is likely that you exhibit that kind of behaviour. Now let us look at what the columns indicate.

Profile

You may have come across the idea of creatures or monkeys sitting on your shoulders. These creatures create dialogue with you and give you internal messages. They talk to you about how you should behave or what you should think. They were put on your shoulders when you were young. Whatever your childhood experiences were, either positive or negative, you were still given early behavioural messages: How to be careful when you crossed the road, what and how to eat, how to dress yourself. There are both positive and negative messages. Some would be positive and helpful like "be happy" but other negative ones may have had long term damaging effects, like you're "stupid", "thick", "no good at sports", "can't draw", "nasty evil person", "waste of space".

As you have matured and been influenced by other factors and people then some of the creatures may have dropped off your shoulders. Nevertheless let us have a look to see if some of them might still be chatting to you.

What do the columns tell you?

Column A – be perfect
Column B – please people
Column C – hurry up
Column D – be strong
Column E – try harder

* If you work through work out 6, you will be able to change your behaviour, release yourself from inner manipulation, your hooks and knock the nasty creatures off your shoulders. When you do this, let's say one a day, keeps submission and depression well at bay.

Personal Psychic Profile
Mind matters
6

1. Are you reluctant to show your feelings? ☐ ☐

2. When setting standards for yourself are they usually too high? ☐ ☐

3. Do you sometimes feel out upon when helping others? ☐ ☐

4. Do you take on too many jobs at the same time? ☐ ☐

5. Do you dislike letting go of a job, thinking with a bit more effort I could improve this task? ☐ ☐

6. Do you like to get things right? ☐ ☐

7. Do you like to be liked preferring to be popular than unpopular? ☐ ☐

8. Do you find it difficult to delegate or ask for help? ☐ ☐

9. Do little things annoy you; a picture not quite straight, a disorderly desk, spelling mistakes? ☐ ☐

10. Do you tend to collect for somebody's present or organize your work special gatherings? ☐ ☐

11. Do you become irritated when someone takes ages to come to the point? ☐ ☐

12. Do you use other people, or their work as a yardstick for your own performance and judge yourself accordingly? ☐ ☐

13. Are you reluctant to give up a job, or stop reading a book, which you are not enjoying? ☐ ☐

14. Do you go to work when you are feeling ill even though others would stay away with the same symptoms? ☐ ☐

15. Do you finish off. Or add to, people's sentences in the hope that they'll get on with it? ☐ ☐

16. Do you like to be organized and keep thing neat and tidy? ☐ ☐

17. Do you hate people wasting time talking about what they might to do, instead of just doing it? ☐ ☐

18. Would you find it difficult to share your personal concerns with someone? ☐ ☐

19. Do you try to avoid conflict so as not to upset other people? ☐ ☐

20. Do you push yourself to achieve a better job or relationship, or to gain more qualifications? ☐ ☐

Complete the following five (A-E), putting your score next to the question numbers below. Give yourself 1 point if you have answered Yes, 0 point if No. Calculate your score for each column.

Column	A	B	C	D	E
Questions	2 ☐	3 ☐	4 ☐	1 ☐	5 ☐
Questions	6 ☐	7 ☐	11 ☐	8 ☐	12 ☐
Questions	9 ☐	10 ☐	15 ☐	14 ☐	13 ☐
Questions	16 ☐	19 ☐	17 ☐	18 ☐	20 ☐

TOTAL ☐ ☐ ☐ ☐ ☐
SCORE ☐ ☐ ☐ ☐ ☐

Assessment: GIVIG AND RECEIVING COMPLIMENTS

Being able to give and receive compliments without embarrassment or denial reflects a healthy level of self-confidence and self-worth. How fit are you at giving and receiving compliment?

Look at the scenarios below. Tick your most likely response.

1. Your books compliment you on a report you have prepared. What do you think, say or do?

    A. Reply 'Thanks, but I don't really think it's that great', or ☐

    B. 'Thank you, that feels good.' ☐

    C. Think to yourself 'What are they after?' ☐

2. David, a joiner member of your team, has just delivered an excellent presentation to one of your clients. What do you think, say or do?

    A. Think to yourself 'keep your hands off, this one's mine!' , or ☐

    B. 'O well, they'll probably want David, not me, to handle their account from now on.' ☐

    C. Walk over and say 'Well done, first-rate presentation. I really think it went down well.' ☐

3. You are congratulated on winning promotion. What do you think, say or do?

    A. Say 'Thanks, I'm absolutely thrilled with the promotion', or ☐

B. 'I should think so too after all the hard work I have put into this company' , or □

C. 'it is a fluke, I don't really deserve it!' □

Personal Psychic Profile
Mind matters
7

Handling Criticism and Emotions.

Liberating language to avoid or handle criticism.

Handling criticism can be easier if you are using appropriate language. Instead of saying, "You make me feel angry when you speak to me like that", say, "I feel angry when you speak to me like that".

Negative feelings can change with positive thoughts. So, thinking of the right words to use will help you be more assertive. For instance, feeling anxious about Information Technology when the words you are hearing are new can create an inner fear. So, learning and understanding specific words will help.

The language people use can directly affect how you react to that person. Many people would object to swearing or defamatory comments about work or home situations, but often it is subtler than that.

Speech might include using certain words that create a feeling of unease in you or you may be using such words that affect how individuals relate to you. For instance, using words like:

* working "for" people, instead of working "with" them;
* battle language like "axe" the expenditure instead of reduce;
* "confront" or "tackle" people instead of "address"
* "problems" instead of "issues" or "concerns"
* "why" instead of "what" or "how";
* "ought" instead of "could"
* "should" instead of "may"
* "coloured" instead of "black".

What words affect you and create negative feelings in you?

Some words are bound to be emotive, like "cancer", but it may be difficult to find a replacement for them. At least think about them. The word "redundancy" can create fear, unless someone is looking forward to retirement, or wanting to change jobs anyway.

As well as the words themselves, there is the way in which you speak. Many people still have misconceptions about the difference between aggressive and assertive language. So you may be using the right words, but speaking in an abrupt, chipped way.

Certain accents and dialects may irritate you. Yours may irritate your staff. You cannot do much about that, but at least be aware that you may be dismissing someone just because of the way they speak.

Personal Psychic Profile
Mind matters
8

Establishing Your Values.

Now look at your list in fitness assessment 9, and see if the same names also appear in assessment 8.

If they do, then put a mark against their name. Any surprises?

Now check to see in which list they appeared, (Were they written in the A or B column, in 10?)

Now analyse the following ten questions from your fitness assessment 9.

1. Did the people you like show up in Column A?

_____

2. Did the people you dislike show up in column B?

_____

3. Did the people you trust show up in Column A?

_____

4. Did the people you distrust show up in column B?

_____

5. Did the people you thought were promoted beyond their ability shows up in column B?

_____

6. Did the people you have negative feelings towards show up in column B?

_____

7. Did the people you have positive feelings towards appear up in column A?

_____

8. Did the people you find sexually attractive show up in column A?

_____

9. Did the people you find intellectually stimulating show up in column A?

_____

10. Did you find the people with a good sense of humour showed up in column A?

_____

Have you found that most of the people you feel positive about appear in column A and those you feel negative towards in column B? Does this tell you anything? See P8 for your prescription to understanding how or why you create a feeling of being ill at ease or non-assertive with yourself, about some people but not with others.

Having answered the questionnaire, consider the following reasons for your responses.

1. ASSERTIVE PEOPLE RECOGNIZE THEIR VALUE SYSTEMS

Who do you like?

People we like usually share our values and belief systems. The name of the person you like probably shares yours, making it highly likely that you will be assertive with them. You probably find this person easier to manage, to be managed by them or to live with them, since you talk the same language or at least share some common values, which makes your starting point that much further along the line when explaining your requirements of them, or issuing them with instructions or discussing new projects and ideas. You are starting from the same point and do not need to battle with trivia. You just know that they understand how, why, or on what basic beliefs your decisions have been made. You are likely to be coming from being mutually supportive, well at least most of the time. This does not mean that you never disagree, but at least there is a common understanding of each other's viewpoint.

2. ASSERTIVE PEOPLE UNDERSTAND THE REASONS FOR NOT ENGAGING WITH EVERYONE.

Who do you dislike?

In contrast, the people you don't like probably do not share your value systems. For example, If they make racist, or sexist remarks, and you hold the concept of the equality of people as a strong value, then these are people with whom you will have difficulties in working or, living, or managing. There are also many other reasons for not liking them. You may just not like their physical appearance or they may remind you of someone similar, whom you didn't like. Or you may see traits in them that you see in yourself. That is, traits that you don't like about yourself. Of course sometimes you may not like them because you believe that they are just not a very genuine person.

You may feel insecure about your own ability and dislike someone who is more capable, more of an academic than yourself, or perhaps they applied for the post you now hold and you still feel guilty that you were chosen in preference to them. They may be giving you non-verbal messages and signs that they are not impressed with your working or management style and that really they could do the job better than you.

3. ASSERTIVE PEOPLE ARE TRUSTING

Who do you trust?

The person you trust has probably shown you their vulnerable side and it is highly likely that you have reciprocated. They probably trust you. Everyone needs support at some time and life may become difficult for you at home with family, friends or at work with your working colleagues. So it is very positive that you have someone with whom you can share confidences in the knowledge that any information given to them will not be disclosed to others.

4. ASSERTIVE PEOPLE ACCEPT THAT IF TRUST IS BROKEN IT DOES NOT RETURN TO THE SAME LEVEL.

Who has broken or betrayed your trust?

Now you have identified someone where trust has been broken, think back to how this happened and how you have managed that relationship since. It is important that you deal with that broken trust that you tell the person how you feel. Once trust has been broken, then no matter how hard you try to re-establish that same trusting relationship, it never reaches the same level. There is always an element of mistrust lingering in the background. Think of someone at work or at home who has broken your trust in him or her. Did you try to work really hard at salvaging the relationship, tried to trust again, but were unable to get back to the security and level of trust that you shared previously? Has that been your experience? Ask yourself what you can do about it. If anything do it, if not then forget it.

5. ASSERTIVE PEOPLE DON'T WASTE THEIR TIME BEING JEALOUS OR ENVIOUS

Who has been promoted beyond their ability?

On what did you base your opinion of someone promoted beyond his or her ability? Perhaps they secured the position for which you applied. Maybe it is pure envy or jealousy. Have they got the ear of someone whom YOU would like to impress, or do you think they were appointed under "suspicious circumstances"? Perhaps they were friends or lovers. Maybe there was a possible collapse of their previous appointment, so a new appointment was bestowed upon them, thus avoiding redundancy. Can you do anything about it? If you can, then do it, if you can't then forget it.

6. ASSERTIVE PEOPLE ARE INTELLECTUALLY STIMULATED

Who stimulates you intellectually?

You are more likely to be assertive with someone who intellectually stimulates you, rather than someone who bores you because you may tend to think that it is not worth bothering to voice your needs.

Do you need to be stimulated in order to work to your full potential? If you need a challenge, then both your right and left-hand brain needs to be encouraged. The right side of the brain is your artistic side; the left side is the factual side. You need to give yourself permission to use both, otherwise you may be right or left-hand side deprived! Spend more time with people who stimulate you intellectually. It is like a tonic and can enable you to grow and move in new ways. Recognize your need for intellectual stimulus.

7. ASSERTIVE PEOPLE CAN LAUGH AT THEMSELVES

Who has a good sense of humour?

Humour can vary with culture, gender, geographical areas, age, sexual orientation, and religion or with specific situations. There can be a lot of "game playing" going on for you at work. Pomposity, arrogance and power games. One of the most useful assets you can have is that of a spontaneous sense of humour. There will be times when you will need to 'loosen up', relax, step back from the pressures and try to see the funny side. Laughter is considered to reduce blood pressure and so help stave off many serious illnesses. So enjoy your work! Laugh, be spontaneous and have some fun in your job.

8. ASSERTIVE PEOPLE ENJOY THEIR SEXUALITY

Who do you find sexually attractive?

Sexuality is all around you both in and out of work! It takes up a lot of psychic energy. Management books do not discuss sexual relationships at work but so much psychic energy is used on such feelings. It is OK to feel sexual to people but it is how you behave that is important. Remember each choice has a consequence. Admitting to yourself how you feel is the first step. You may find it more difficult to be assertive with someone that you sexually attracted towards. But go on try it. After all most people are more attracted to assertive people rather than to wimps or bullies.

9. ASSERTIVE PEOPLE FEEL POSITIVE

Who do you have positive feelings towards?

When you have positive feelings towards a certain individual, you are likely to feel comfortable in their company. You may be projecting the positive feelings onto that person that you have had towards someone else in your life.

10. ASSERTIVE PEOPLE OVERCOME THEIR NEGATIVITY BY REALIZING THAT THEY ARE AS GOOD AS EVERYONE ELSE.

Who do you have negative feelings towards?

I have left this question until the last because it probably causes you more problems than the others! Feeling negative towards someone is not the best basis for being assertive either in a working relationship or any other personal relationship. So start now by loving yourself.

Personal Psychic Profile
Mind matters
9

Your Rights

How did you score?

Write down the statements that you did not tick in your fitness assessment number

....

....

....

....

What are your reasons for believing that you do not have the above, listed rights?

....

....

....

....

What do you think that you could do about to believe that you do have such rights?

....

....

....

....

26. How Assertive Are You?

Your mind is powerful. Remember how you think affects how you feel and behave. Your mind can help you to live a more fulfilling happy life and look after your emotional needs. I hope that you find one thought that you think is helpful to you.

Assertive behaviour is about being honest, open and direct. When we are assertive, we feel grounded, focused, and able to ask for what we want or need. At the same time, we need to recognise that others also have their needs.

Assertiveness is often confused with being aggressive and appeasing behaviour as being shy and quiet.

So what do you gain or lose, by being assertive?

You gain:
Self-love, improved self-worth
Self-confidence
Inner harmony
Improved quality of life
Real intimacy
Caring friends
Trust
Respect
Influence
Genuine game free honest relationships

What do you lose? Nothing!

What can you gain or lose from being Non-Assertive?

You gain:
A quiet life
Avoidance of conflict
Control of inner feelings
Praise for conforming.
Depression
Psychosomatic illness.

You lose:
Self-love
Confidence
The ability to clear the atmosphere of conflict
The respect of others
The power to make decisions
The satisfaction of being mentally intimate
Succeeding in relationships
Psychosomatic wellness

Now look for the activities and exercises that will build your fitness:

1. BEHAVING ASSERTIVELY THROUGH THINKING AND FEELING POSITIVE

1. You may choose to start by realizing that you can say no. With practise later you will learn to say "no" without feeling guilty.

2. You are allowed to make mistakes, so admit it. You may use humour to quell a critical situation by saying "That's the first mistake I've made in my life".

3. You can ask for what you want recognising others have needs too. People cannot read your mind so tell them what you are thinking.

4. Say, "I need to think that over". The word "I" gives you power.

I feel hurt when you treat me in that way.

NOT

You make me feel hurt – that gives your power away to the other person.

5. Express your feelings, avoid turning them inward. In-turned, frozen anger can lead to depression.

6. Accept yourself and

Give yourself permission to grieve or to be angry or to be ill. Avoid trying to be Wonder Woman or Superman.

7. Use assertive language – I wish to say – I believe – I think and feel, I need to listen,

NOT

"Can I just say"; "Can I add to what you've just said".

It rings of permission seeking like "Can I just have a little breathe of your air".

8. Be assertive about your worth. Look after yourself emotionally, physically and mentally.

Take selfish time and enjoy it, treat yourself to small luxuries and rebuild your self-esteem. Take exercise, relaxation, stand upright, and eat sensibly.

9. Smile when you want to, not because you think you have to do, in order that people will like you. Remember:

Powerful people smile when please.

Powerless people smile to please.

10. So try changing your behaviour, remember:

"If you always do what you've always done, You'll always get what you've always got". So try something different.

Try this list.

One a day – Keeps submission and depression at bay.

PERSONAL PSYCHIC PROFILE

So you've had your fitness check-up and identified your strengths and weaknesses. Now is the time to take action!

Packed with practical exercises and activities, the Workout contains almost all the equipment you need to become super fit at assertiveness.

Look back it your personal fitness profile. Where do your strengths and weaknesses lie? Did they lie in specific areas of the skill-are you, for example, generally strong when it comes to getting things done, but weak when it comes to managing conflict? Or do they lie across all three skills areas? Depending on your personal fitness profile, you can either focus on improving the particular area of skill, or work on individual weaknesses within each area.

Of course, if you want to raise your level of performance in all areas, complete all the activities, then you really will be super fit!

Work-outs 1 2 and 3 relate directly to fitness profile 1, 2 and 3.

Similarly, work-outs 4-7 and 8-10.

Personal Psychic Profile
1

Self-Confidence Feelings and Emotions

"If you always do what you've always done, you'll always get what you've always got."

So, try something different.

Self-confidence is the key to behaving assertively. To build up your self-confidence you need to think and feel positively. The following will help you to build your self-confidence.

To be physically fit, you need to start from within. Eating the correct foods, digesting and excreting your rubbish. So, it is the same with working out on your self-confidence.

- Taking in the correct thoughts,
- Digesting or internalising them and

- Eliminating your rubbish.

What follows are some of the correct ways of thinking, try to internalise them, think about them and accept them as being pertinent to you. You may have been subjected to a great deal of rubbish over your lifetime but that does not mean that you have to still carry it about with you.

By trying out some of the following exercises you will create your own fitness pack. It is like having your very own personal trainer. So try changing your behaviour, remember:

Try out some of the ideas on this list;

One a day, keeps submission at bay.

* You may choose to start by realizing that you can say no. With practise, later you will learn to say "no" without feeling guilty.
* You are allowed to make mistakes, so admit it. You may use humour to quell a critical situation by saying "That's the first mistake I've made in my life".
* You can ask for what you want but also recognize that others have needs too.
* People cannot read your mind so tell them what you are thinking.
* Also recognize that you can say, "I need to think that over". The word "I" gives you power.
* Use assertive language – I wish to say – I believe – I think and feel, I need to listen,

NOT

"Can I just say"; "Can I add to what you've just said".

It rings of permission seeking like "Can I just have a little breathe of your air".

* Be assertive about your worth. Look after yourself emotionally, physically and mentally.

Take selfish time and enjoy it, treat yourself to small luxuries and rebuild your self-esteem. Take exercise, relaxation, stand upright, and eat sensibly.

* You might find it easier to do if you digest the tips from the trainer.
* Express your feelings and avoid turning them inward. In-turned, frozen anger can lead to depression.

Say "I feel hurt when you treat me in that way."

NOT

"You make me feel hurt", as that gives your power away to the other person.

* Accept yourself and give yourself permission to grieve or to be angry or to be ill. Avoid trying to be Wonder Woman or Superman.
* Smile when you want to, not because you think you have to do, in order that people will like you. Remember:

Powerful people smile when please.
Powerless people smile to please.

Personal Psychic Profile
2

1. GIVING AND RECEIVING COMPLIMENTS, WORK OUT.

How many times has someone said to you 'I like your hair' and you, with a toss of your hand, pushing it back, have replied 'It needs washing!' Or to 'I like your tie' responded with 'what was wrong with the one that I wore yesterday'. So it is important to be able to assertively accept compliments and not to 'discount' the other person's feelings or thoughts.

Now to do your practical work-out.

Complete the following exercise by ticking the relevant box:

Before my fitness programme, I found it;

Easy to accept compliments; _____

Embarrassing, when given compliments _____

Difficult to accept compliments; _____

Awkward to know what to say, when complimented; _____

What would you now reply to the following comments? _____

Your partner compliments you on your appearance.

_____

Your friend has just met your new partner. How do you respond when they tell you that they think he or she is terrific?

_____

I used to only give compliments to,

_____

Now I am able to,

_____

You are congratulated on your successful results at work; for example, a super sale; an examination; with a new contract; completing a project on time.

_____

Now, my personal trainer has helped me to realize that,

_____

_____

2. GIVING AN RECEIVING FEEDBACK

Now to do your practical work-out.

Complete the following exercise by ticking the relevant box:

Before my fitness programme, I found it;

Easy to accept compliments; _____

Embarrassing, when given compliments; _____

Difficult to accept compliments; _____

Awkward to know what to say, when complimented; _____

What would you now reply to the following comments? _____

Your partner compliments you on your appearance.

_____

Your friend has just met your new partner. How do you respond when they tell you that they think he or she is terrific?

_____

I used to only give compliments to,

_____

Now I am able to,

_____

You are congratulated on your successful results at work; for example, a super sale; an examination; with a new contract; completing a project on time.

_____

Now, my personal trainer has helped me to realize that,

_____

_____

Personal Psychic Profile

3

THE BODY IMAGE WORK OUT

Having worked out some of the possible perceptions that people may make when listening to your body talk, now you need to work out are exactly what you need to do in order to present an assertive image to others.

How fit is your body when communicating with other people?

Your body talks! It tells people what you are feeling or thinking.

In order to feel fit you need to begin by checking up on what you think you or others are saying when they adopt certain body postures.

Test it out.

Begin by looking at the following illustrations and write down what you are feeling or thinking about a person if they were to use such a gesture.

(ARMS CROSSED)   (LEGS CROSSED)

(POINTED FINGER)   (STEEPLED HANDS)

(FOOT UP)   (TWIRLING HAIR)

(ARMS BEHIND HEAD)   (HANDS ON MOUTH)

(EYES LOWERED)   (SITTING FORWARD)

Now look at your fitness profile, in order to see how fit you are, in terms of your body talk. Discover how you could look, which can strongly depend on how you are feeling. In fact so much non-assertive behaviour is based on your lack of inner fitness.

Your feelings can be communicated in so many different ways. Your body talk may be interpreted as aggressive, avoiding, adaptive or appeasing. When really you need to be being perceived as assertive.

In order to feel fit you need to communicate being assertive.

Even though inwardly you may feel nervous or anxious about a certain person or in a certain situation.

Presenting Yourself

Remember there are cultural differences in different parts of the world. Some of the gestures I refer to are multi-cultural, others may just belong to the Western world. For example, people of different nationalities may have different personal spaces. Some people will naturally move very close to the person to whom they are speaking, whereas in some countries, outside Britain, this may be regarded as not very acceptable behaviour. As might, for instance, showing the under sole of your shoe or looking into the eyes of someone older or wiser than yourself. Also within the same culture, there will be some people who have differing preferences of body gestures. For instance, some individuals like to be touched, whereas others will shy away from physical contact of any kind.

Assertive body language

When someone talks to you, you are only hearing a small percentage of what they are actually saying, but you are picking up a greater percentage of information through the messages which are being given to you by their body movements. You may be doing this unconsciously, but nevertheless it is affecting how you are thinking or feeling about that person. For example, saying something positive to someone, but also pointing your finger will be picked up as aggressive and critical rather than praise.

So your prescription is to be aware of how the different parts of your body can talk to others.

Now look in the mirror and check out the following pointers.

Head talk

The nodding of the head almost universally indicates "Yes", or agreement, whereas the shaking of the head implies the opposite, that is, refusing or disagreeing.

When people are happy, they smile: when they are miserable, they frown or grimace.

Facial expressions are particular give-aways:

The raising of an eyebrow may indicate puzzlement.

The raising of the forehead might be amazement or disbelief.

Eye talk

It is thought that:

* most right-handed people will raise their eyes to the left, (as you are looking at them) if they are to recall incidents…
* to the right when creating images…
* look straight at you when listening.
* lower the eyes when into emotions or feelings.

Of course, some people could still be listening to you with their eyes lowered, because what is being said between you is creating a set of positive or negative emotions in them.

146

The raising of the eyes to the left or to the right is reversed by 6% of the population. Many of the people in this group are left-handed, but not all. So in some cases the eyes move in the opposite direction to that which has been described.

Face talk

It is not only movements of the face but also the movements of the hands on the face that may indicate when somebody is lying:

* The hand across the mouth;
* The finger on the lip: perhaps not wanting to disclose.
* Lifting the hands above the shoulders and around the face can also de-power you, like fiddling with hair
* Stroking a beard
* Or sucking your glasses, may again take away your power. The sucking of glasses is also supposed to indicate that you are waiting for time or silently requesting "thinking it over" time.

Shoulder talk

Universally the shoulder shrug... is accepted as:

* "I don't quite understand"
* "I don't really know what you are talking about"
* If the shoulders are lifted with tension around them, then this may indicate fear. (We lodge fear in our shoulders, anger in our calves, and supposedly sexual problems in the lower back).

Arm talk if the arms are folded, then this may indicate;

* That you want to block somebody out or
* Feeling uncomfortable with yourself or the situation you are in. Many people will say, "I only cross my arms like this because it makes me feel more comfortable." And they are right, because when we are feeling uncomfortable, we give ourselves a little cuddle.

Touch talk

What a lot of information about you can be gleaned from touch! The most likely tactile interaction you will have with someone is probably going to be a handshake.

You can have an appeasing, submissive handshake, where the palm is uppermost or,

An aggressive, dominant handshake, where the palm is lowered over and on top of the other people.

So, to be assertive, remember that the shaking of the hand can create a tremendous impression on your first meeting with someone.

If you are shaking hands, then shake hands with your hand as far up to the other person's thumb as you possibly can. Shake firmly, as there is nothing worse than a limp, wet-trout handshake!

Equally, it is just as off-putting if you are shaking hands with a vice-like grip that almost cuts rings into your victim's fingers!

Then there is the gloved handshake where someone will put both their hands around yours, shaking with one and covering the back of your palm with their other hand. This may make people feel smothered or intimidated.

In some countries people may hold your elbow whilst shaking your hand, or hold your wrist or even the upper arm, or shoulder hold.

So, give a positive assertive handshake.

Hand talk

If somebody is sitting with their elbows on the table and their hands inter-twined, blocking their body, this can indicate;

* A tendency to hold in negative feelings, even though they may be smiling.
* Inter-twined hands indicate resistance.
* Open hands show acceptance.
* The higher the hands are held, the more resistant the person is, however, clenched hands held low down the body, would still tend keep people at bay.

Then there is the "steepling" of hands, the "raised steeple" would indicate;

* A superior to a subordinate interaction, a kind of know-it-all, patronizing or confident attitude.

Ear talk

The ear-rub may be indicating that;

* You really don't want to hear any more, or
* You have heard enough and would like to talk yourself.

Next talk

The neck-scratch is supposed to indicate;

* "I don't know if that is correct, really".

Then there is the collar-pull.

Desmond Morris found that when people were lying there was a tingling sensation around the face and neck tissues, which needed to be rubbed or scratched to ease it. This may also be the case when somebody is angry or frustrated and needs to pull their collar away from their neck. Of course, it could just mean that they are hot, or that the collar is uncomfortable!

Leg talk

As well as crossing arms, many people cross their legs. This may be perceived as pushing people, even though you may feel very comfortable, the other person to is likely to feel uncomfortable.

but again it is useful to realize that it is not what you think you are saying with your body, but what is being picked up by the messages you are sending out.

If you cross your arms and legs:

* You look as though it is going to be very difficult for someone to convince you of what they are trying to say to you. Or you are actually showing displeasure before, or during, the conversation.
* Cross your legs and, or, hold on to your leg as a barrier, like a kind of

arm-lock or leg-lock;

* This position would mean that you are rather stubborn, or tough minded, and it is going to be very difficult to break through your present attitude.

Sit talk

How you sit will be giving off all kinds of messages. There are conflicting thoughts about someone who sits with their arms behind their heads. Either,

* You come across as "One day you will be as intelligent as I am", or,
* You look so laid-back that you don't appear to be taking anything too seriously that is being said to you.
* Where you sit on the chair can indicate various things. If you lean forward:
* Then this is an invasion of the others space.
* You look as if you are ready to finish talking to them.
* I you sit with one arm just hooked on the back of a chair, this may be giving the impression of;
* "I really don't want to be here".
* Of course, very few of you would sit with your feet up on the desk, I hope but if so;
* This would be about ownership and claiming your territory.
* If you are relaxed enough to sit with one leg over the arm of a chair... then,
* You really are coming over as someone who hasn't got a great deal of concern for what is being said to you.

Finger talk

Then there is the pointed finger. If you point your finger at people, you must be being critical; and it looks aggressive not assertive. You cannot say anything supportive and helpful if your finger is wagging. Some people may know better than to actually point a finger, but instead they will use a pen, or anything else that is likely to be dictatorial, to emphasise the message they are delivering.

Foot talk

Finally, the big give-away is the feet. If you turn your foot up:

* Then this would indicate that you are uncomfortable, either with the question you have just been asked or with what is being talked about. This gesture is called "crying with the feet". In fact, so much knowledge can be gained by learning how to interpret the signals transmitted by people's feet, that it really is amazing that everyone doesn't know all about it!

So, your prescription is to be aware that there may be many reasons for people moving their bodies in certain ways. If you want to be assertive then a good rule of thumb is to sit in an "open" body position whilst keeping as still as you possibly can, this will make the other person feel more relaxed and comfortable in your presence. Recognise that your "body talk" may well be sending out negative messages, which could be entirely opposite to those which you intended. If you think this applies to you, then remember that your prescriptive Golden Rule one is to "Fake it till you make it".

Golden Rule two is to "Create Rapport"

How Can I Create Rapport?

RAPPORT is spelt RAP ORT

Sixty to eighty percent of human communication is done non-verbally (Allan Pease 1993).

When talking to people with whom you feel comfortable, you are likely to demonstrate this ease by your body gestures. The converse is true. Consider the following suggestions, and remember, it is not what you think you are communicating, it is what people are seeing and receiving that gets your message across.

If you are assertive then you will gel. If you don't gel then it is likely to be because you are missing a vital ingredient, that is, rapport. If you haven't got rapport you haven't got anything!

Assertive rapport enables you to put people at their ease, gives you an instant insight into how they are feeling, enables you to communicate more effectively, generating a feeling of warmth, even trust. And the good news is that with a little effort on your part you can go a long way towards acquiring this skill!

* Keep as attentive as possible and sit facing the person,
* Readily accepting eye contact.

* Keep your body language open.
* Try to use the same tone or speed of voice when talking with someone.

This can be difficult between genders, but none the less it is possible. If someone is speaking very quickly and you speak very slowly, then there is likely to be little rapport. Also, if they have a high-pitched voice and yours is very low and deep, then there will be little rapport. This is not to say you should mimic the other person, but be aware of slightly modulating your tone and speed as best you can. When people have rapport, often you will hear their voice tones change in essence with each other.

Apart from your voice, there is also the aspect of the language that you use. If you are talking to someone and ask them;

"What do you think about…" and they reply;

"Well, I feel that…" then you are likely to think that they are not answering your question.

Equally, if you are asked a question and omit to use their language, then they may think that you don't understand, or you are not on their same wavelength.

SELF CONFIDENCE CHECK LIST

In which situations am I assertive?

_____

In which situations am I either appeasing or aggressive?

_____

WITH WHOM DO I WORK WELL?

List the names of three people with whom you work, who would fall into one of the two following categories. Try to put three into each column. If you cannot think of three, then it does not matter; simply write down as many as you can.

PEOPLE WITH WHOM:

A: I WORK WELL   **B:** DO NOT WORK WELL

....

....

....

REASONS FOR COLUMN A

_____

_____

REASONS FOR COLUMN B

_____

_____

People with whom I find it difficult to state my beliefs

_____

_____

Because

_____

People that I would really love to be able to tell, what I really think of them

_____

_____

People that I believe have overlooked my ability

_____

Reasons.

_____

Before reading this book, I found it:

- easy to accept compliments   _____
- embarrassing when given compliments   _____

- difficult to accept compliments   _____
- awkward to know what to say, when complimented   _____

Now, I have learned that

_____

_____

_____

What would you *now* reply to the following comments?

1. Your partner compliments you on your appearance.

_____

_____

_____

2. Your friend has just met your new partner. How do you respond when they tell you that they think he or she is terrific?

_____

_____

_____

3. You are congratulated on your successful results; for example, on an examination; dinner party; driving test; a new project or sporting event.

_____

_____

_____

I used to only give compliments to

_____

Now I am able to give compliments to

_____

Look at the following ten pointers, check which you do:

                                                  Yes   No

1. Shaking hands firmly, not aggressively.

2. Smiling only when genuinely pleased.

3. Keeping your arms below your shoulders.

4. Uncrossing your legs.

5. Placing your feet firmly on the floor.

6. Unfolding your arms.

7. Relaxing your hands.

8. Having an open, accepting body posture.

9. Keeping still as stillness is empowering.

10. Holding your head at the same angle as the person to whom you are speaking.

Personal Psychic Profile 4

Getting Things Done

THE WORK OUT AT MEETINGS

The purpose meetings is to get things done, so first of all ask yourself, "Is this meeting really necessary?"

There are three things to consider in meetings, the three "P's"

Product   Process   People

Exchange Ideas to Achieve 'Win-Win'

The skills of negotiating are very easy for some, but very difficult for others.

People may have different needs.

Some of your staff need explanations.

Tell your staff the reasons why.

Fantasy is often worse than reality. Once they know your reasoning, they are more likely to feel inclined to go along with you.

If you want to appear more assertive at meetings – try out these tips.

* Speak out early, even if it is only to say, "Good Morning". So that you don't end up thinking "I'm the only one who hasn't spoken so far" and getting yourself into an anxious state.

* This is the reverse behaviour of the aggressive person who loves to hear the sound of his or her own voice. They are predictable in voicing

their opinions with the result that people often psychologically switch off.

* Keep contributions short.
* Avoid interrupting others and don't let others interrupt you.
* Keep non-verbal behaviour assertive.
* Time your contributions.
* Get a reaction to your contribution.
* It is fine to change your mind.
* Make at least one positive contribution, even if it is just agreeing. This is active rather than passive agreement.
* Request the reasons for any changes. For instance, a cut in staffing.
* Ask for clarification if anything seems unclear. It is a good sign that you are listening to the arguments and still engaged in the debate.
* Express your feelings, although other people may find your anger difficult to handle.
* Remember that if you've been invited to join a meeting, you have equal rights to be heard, seen and respected.
* When speaking, you have the right to being heard without interruption.
* Assertive people say, "I don't understand". By saying this it is likely that others will both warm towards you and agree with you when you have been braving enough to say what you are thinking.
* Avoid worrying about sounding stupid, and say so if you don't really understand or agree with something.
* Aggressive behaviour is likely to lose you support.
* Don't be afraid to checkout if other people agree or disagree with what is being said.
* Ask for feedback by asking the others at the meeting for their reaction to your ideas.
* Always check out what people think they then have to go away and do.
* When writing up minutes of a meeting, be brief, with the initials of the person designated to action the suggestions.

Personal Psychic Profile 5

SAYING 'NO'

So in order to be assertive and to be able to say 'no', you need to recognise how to use language in a way that positively expresses what you are really wanting. That is not saying 'Yes' when you really mean 'No'.

This means that you do not become pulled down avenues into which you do not want to go, resulting in a labyrinth of irrelevant argument. So you need to continue to make your point.

* 'No I am unable to do that.' You can add sorry if you want to but try to just say the word 'No'.

* Remember to repeat your core phrase. "What I need from you is."

* Consider your basic needs. Do not ask for what you want, but what you need. You may want a lot of money, but exactly how much do you need? Be sure to be specific, so instead of saying "I want you to work professionally", a basic need would be to start with specifically would be "What I need from you is for you to be on time".

* Demonstrate that you are hearing what the other person is saying. "Yes, I do realize that you have personal problems at home, however, 'No' I cannot change the agreed arrangements".

* Empathise with the other person about their situation, understanding their frame of reference as to what they are saying to you. For example, "That is sounding very difficult for you and I recognise that it will be creating pressure on you, however, 'No' I cannot help".

* Recognise your fallback position as to how far you are prepared to alter your needs according to the other person's wishes. This will help you to avoid being pushed further back from your own targets.

Personal Psychic Profile 6

DEALING WITH MANIPULATION

Ancestral voices or early childhood messages, are like little creatures that sit on your shoulder and can create non-assertive behaviour. You need to become aware of them and remove them in order to feel fit.

They are also referred to as:

PSYCHOLOGICAL DRIVERS
The Be Perfect person or manager:

You may have heard jokes about different kinds of managers:-

Mushroom management – keeps people in the dark. Every now and again throws a load of manure on to them!

Kipper management – two faced and spineless!

Seagull management – hovering above and then swooping down and dropping rubbish from a great height upon you!

Goldfish management – the dead rise to the top!

Diamond room management – this is the equivalent of the 'Be Perfect' person or manager.

The diamond room person lives in a room full of diamonds, diamond ceiling, floor and walls. Yet right in the corner is a load of manure. Instead of seeing the diamonds around you, you focus on the manure. Similarly, you might find yourself concentrating on the small percentage of things that are wrong with an individual instead of celebrating the diamonds in their make-up.

You may play the psychological game of 'blemish' which again is looking for the mistake rather than appreciating the whole. For instance someone hands you a finished project and your first reaction is one of "There's a spelling mistake on page 90" instead of saying assertively, "Thank you there's a lot of good work gone into this. However, I am concerned about one or two small spelling mistakes, let's get those right."

The Pleasing People person

Well if you have found this creature chatting to you then you will probably nod a lot and smile a lot at people. Even when you don't agree with them or feel upset.

You are probably liked but may come over as pretty ineffectual when it comes to sorting out conflict issues.

When you were small you were likely to be told to think about what the neighbours would say, be nice to people. The message that you were picking up is that unless you are pleasant to people you are no good. Somehow you will be punished. So your style is to make others feel good so you can feel better. You find it really difficult to say 'No'.

The Hurry Up person

Gosh everything is such a rush for you. You are always busy doing so many things simultaneously. Hurrying here hurrying there but still thinking about what else you ought to be doing instead. When you are in a meeting you think about whom you need to speak to at lunch and after work. When you are at lunch you are thinking about being back in the meeting. You probably tap your fingers or twitch your leg more than most. Your speed is admirable but how are the people around you affected. They try to stop you in the corridor but you are in a hurry "I'll see you later" is your reply, but "later" you're just as busy.

It is likely that you arrive late for meetings, letting everyone know how busy you've been. You can irritate others in a meeting with your inability to listen and reflect.

The Be Strong person

You hardly ever have time off work and go in even when you are ill whilst others are off sick with the same condition. Not you. You're there rain or shine in sickness and in health, never recognising when you're tired or hungry, keeping going. You wait until the weekend or holidays to be ill.

The Try Harder person

If you have found that your internal dialogue is about trying harder then you are likely to be always searching for something else. Just take stock of what is good about this job, this relationship. Ask yourself 'For whom am I trying harder?' You may always be looking to the future so you need to ask for what you want now.

You probably share values with some of your staff but also behaviour. Do you get on better with people that share your values or behave like you?

Refer to fitness profile number 10 where you listed 'who works well'. Do any of those names have the same monkeys or creatures on their shoulders, as you have on yours?

GETTING THINGS DONE SECTION CHECKLIST

MEETINGS

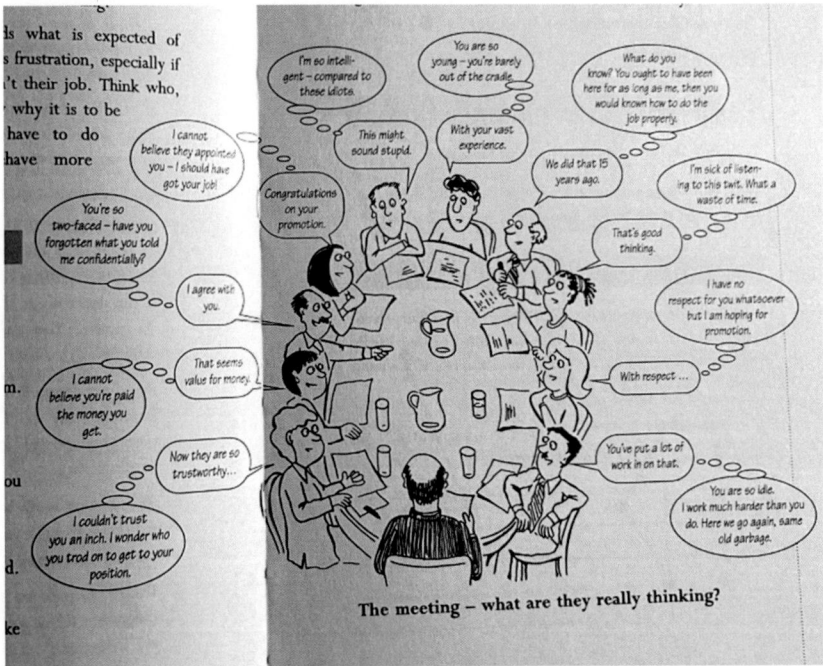

The meeting – what are they really thinking?

What are they really thinking?

I have learned about how I behave in meetings:

_____

How others behave in meetings:

_____

Check out which of the following ideas you will now do to be more assertive in meetings:

	Yes	No

Speak our early in the meeting, if only to say "Hello"
Say when I don't understand
Reflect upon what I think I have heard people saying and ask if it is correct

Request people keep to the point or address the issue being discussed

Use my body gestures to show acceptance or assertive disagreement

Ask people to chat over disagreements later and report back

Listen and express the hidden agendas that I am hearing

Say "Please be brief" or "make a statement" or "What is the point that you are making?"

Avoid saying "With respect" or "Can I just say" instead say "I wish to say" or "I think or feel that"

Say what I think and not expect others to read my mind

Check out that people know what they need to do when they leave the meeting

Write up action points by whom not long, copious minutes.

SAYING NO

To whom do I think I can now say 'No'?
My partner?
My children?
A relative?

A friend?

An employer?

An employee?

A teacher? a doctor? a police officer?

A sales clerk?

Other individuals, give name if you wish?

What could I now say to the following requests?

Also, in which of the following requests of me, could I now say 'No'?

Asking for co-operation from my partner, children, friends, employers, or employees?

_____

A loan of money or of an item?

_____

A favour?

_____

A job?

_____

Love and attention?

_____

Directions?

_____

Others types of requests of me?

_____

When I am with someone who holds a diametrically opposing view to mine, I now think that I could say 'No', if they ask me if I agree with their opposing view on any of the following topics?

Sexual orientation?   Politics?

Racial equality?   Feminism?

My mistakes?   Abortion?

Other's follies?   Other's mistakes?

Capital punishment?   My accomplishments?

Expressing their dislike of a friend of mine?

It can be difficult to be assertive if you are trying to please people, for instance.

The creatures that I found on my shoulder, that is, ancestral voices that create inner talking, were saying:

Be perfect   Please others   Hurry up

Be strong   Try harder

I imbibed these "messages" from

_____

Having identified them I now realize that I can:

_____

What I can specifically do from now on is:

_____

Personal Psychic Profile 7

MANAGING CONFLICT

On the whole almost everyone dislikes conflict. But resolving it assertively can bring positive outcomes.

People can use up your psychic energy both at home and at work. Get your 'people skills' right and the rest of your job becomes easier. You and your colleagues, family and friends will relate more positively, which in turn will bring joy into your home life and workplace. We spend such a large part of our life at work: enjoying work means enjoying life!

Being assertive can mean being a saint, as it is likely that you are expected to manage a variety of people in a fair, unbiased, just and consistent way.

The people with whom you work probably range from the very interesting to the incredibly boring; the intelligent to the stupid; the energised to the fatigued; the old to the young; the motivated to the demotivated and from the genuine to the phoney. They are likely to come from different social, economic and educational backgrounds, have different personalities, values, strengths, goals, needs, abilities and aspirations. What a range! And yet you have to command all your necessary assertive skills in order to manage such diversity.

What is more, even if you are able to be assertive with someone, they could behave differently at other times because of personal issues or concerns, yet you are still expected to manage them, regardless of your own background and needs.

You are expected at all times to be fair, and to work without being prejudice. Yet I guess that there are times when you are prejudiced, when you do pre-judge as to how a person will act or respond to your requests. It is difficult to live or work in harmony, with people when they are aggressive.

Whilst you are expected to be fair, it is likely that there are occasions when you are unfair, when you do give more time to the people you like, or perceivably give more exciting or fulfilling jobs to you favourites.

When you have staff that are not performing up to the standards you expect, then it is imperative that you address these situations. You will need courage, but it will pay off. Hence you will have to consider the question: "Is it because they can't, or is it because they won't?" Hopefully, you will be able to access on what evidence you reached your decision. Also, you may recognize what possible organisational causes may exacerbate unproductive behaviour.

Furthermore, you are likely to recognize the difference between staff who are incompetent or incapable and those who you may need to be disciplined. So you need to ask yourself; '

Is it because they can't or is it because they won't?'

Personal Psychic Profile 8

HANDLING CRITICISM

Regardless of how senior or junior, your position is at work, you will have to manage yourself in order to assertively work with others.

Let us begin by highlighting your relationships with people at work. Forget for a moment what you have to manage and concentrate on whom you have to manage or on who manages you. You only have so much energy and time and it is likely that you are spending an inordinate, disproportional amount of time on some staff rather than on others. Your psychic energy level (that is, the amount of energy you use on psychological thinking or worrying about things) is lowered.

You are highly likely to work or play with a mixture of people, some you like, some you don't, some of whom get on with the job, take up little of your time, to whom you can responsibly delegate and who appear to be successfully achieving their targets.

Whilst others seem to always want to talk to you about inconsequential minute details, fall behind on deadlines, lack drive or sparkle and seem to be take up so much of your precious time. It is likely that you will always have such a mixture, but with astute assertive skills you can help some of the people from the latter group into the former one.

Regardless of these two categories, there is probably something more fundamental going on in you. Something, which you may be reluctant to discuss with others. Thoughts, feelings, emotions and attitudes that you hold towards individuals in both groups.

So, let us explore what it is about you and others that can lead to your being non-assertive that is either appeasing or aggressive, with some people, whilst having the skills and the ability to be assertive and effectively work with others.

Therefore, the first stage is to try to identify what is happening for you emotionally. How you are feeling about the people with whom you work.

Whether they are people you manage or those who manage you. Then the next stage will be to identify what it is about you that may be creating some of the difficulties that you are encountering.

It probably comes down to very basic needs that you have. Maybe you need to be liked, be right, be quick, be strong, or be seen to be in charge and always trying harder. Whatever drives you will have a knock-on effect on those that you manage.

Perhaps you work with some staff, both senior and junior to yourself, whom you think have been promoted beyond their ability. Whilst there are likely to be other people with whom you work where you feel positive, enjoy their company, think that they are a "good laugh", even possibly feel sexually attracted towards them or intellectually stimulated by them.

Now work out on how you can be assertive when criticised?

Virtually every one is criticised from time to time. In order to deal with criticism assertively – first ask yourself:

Is the criticism valid or invalid?

If it is:

Valid   Invalid

Agree with it:

- Say that it's invalid and say why
- Ask for specific times or examples
- Ask yourself who's got the problem.
- You could answer "I can see that's a problem for you!"

How to Criticise Others Assertively

- Tell them what it is that annoys you.
- Tell them how you feel.
- Say what you need, e.g.:
- What I have observed… (is that you shout when I try to discuss our relationship)
- That makes me feel… (rejected and frightened)
- What I need is… (for us to discuss calmly what we are going to do about our money problem.)

- Say "I" to empower yourself,
- Say "Observe" so that they know that you have noticed, not necessarily been told by somebody else.
- Say how you "feel" because people cannot argue with how you feel but they can argue with how you think.
- Say what you "need" otherwise you just go round in circles arguing and justifying, rather than resolving the issue. You may want a great deal but fine it down to a specific need. Avoid saying floppy things like 'I need you to be more professional'. What does that actually mean to someone? Instead be specific like 'I need you to be here on time.'

Personal Psychic Profile 9

ESTABLISHING YOUR VALUES

"SHADOWING" EXERCISES

The following exercises are to enable you to identify with whom you might be subconsciously relating to, when you have strong negative or positive feelings. Think of someone that you feel negative about. Now ask yourself the following questions:

Exercise (1)

WHO DO THEY REMIND ME OF?   _____

(John? Mary? Mother? Head teacher? My first boss? etc.)

Write in the name that comes to mind.

_____

If they do not remind you of anyone go straight to Exercise 2

IN WHAT WAYS IS THIS PERSON LIKE (John etc.)?

Write in the way they are similar and the feelings that occur to you. For example,

Same age? Beard? Looks at me in the same way?   _____

Feel sexually threatened? Sexually excited?   _____

Makes me feel scared, put down or inferior?   _____

Has power over me?   _____

IN WHAT WAYS IS THE PERSON NOT LIKE (John, Mary, etc.)?

Taller? More intelligent? Sense of humour? Different job? We only meet at work, etc. (Put in all the details however trivial they may seem.)

_____

_____

_____

Exercise (2)

This exercise enables you to find out who the person is that is unconsciously affecting you and creating either the negative or positive feelings you have towards them.

HOW DOES THIS PERSON MAKE ME FEEL?

(Angry? Hurt? Excited? One feeling is sufficient)

Write in the feeling

_____

_____

_____

WHO ELSE IN MY LIFE HAS MADE ME FEEL? (Angry etc.)

(Use the word you have used when asking the question)

Write in the name of a person who has also made you feel the same way.

_____

_____

_____

Now you know who they remind you of, complete the rest of the exercise:

WHO DO THEY REMIND ME OF?

_____

_____

_____

(John? Mary? Mother? Head teacher? My first boss? etc.)

Write in the name that comes to mind. If they do not remind you of anyone go straight to next exercise.

IN WHAT WAYS IS THIS PERSON LIKE (John etc.)?

Write in the way they are similar and the feelings that occur to you. For example, Same age? Beard? Looks at me in the same way?

_____

Feel sexually threatened? Sexually excited?

_____

Makes me feel scared, put down or inferior?

_____

Has power over me?

_____

IN WHAT WAYS IS THE PERSON NOT LIKE (John, Mary, etc.)?

Taller? More intelligent? Sense of humour? Different job? We only meet at work, etc. (Put in all the details however trivial they may seem.)

_____

Explanation:

By going through either or both of these exercises you make the "shadow" change into a mosaic pattern, which then fragments and falls away from the person. This enables you to relate to the "shadowless" person more effectively.

You will find this invaluable for clearing your thinking and being able to recognize that often you have difficulty in relating, rather than your colleague, who is probably unaware of how you feel towards him or her. Interestingly, if you feel uncomfortable with someone, for whatever reason, they are likely to feel the same.

So now you can probably identify why you feel negative towards certain people, your line manager, other managers or staff for whom you have some line managerial responsibility.

When you do identify people's "shadows" then it helps to tell the individual something like "you know you just remind me of my father, so sometimes you may find me responding to him rather than you". This can be said in jest, but actually it is helping you to rid yourself of the unnecessary baggage which you are carrying around. Having looked at what might be happening to you in your different working relationships, the next chapter offers you the chance to identify what might be going wrong and how to rectify the situation. We then move on to caring skills, followed by tips on how to deal with conflict, and finally a chapter looking at ways of resolving some contentious situations.

If you are having difficulty relating to someone and experiencing negative feelings but cannot clearly see or understand why this is the case, then consider "shadowing" as a possible cause. This means that some people may have a "shadow" of someone else you have known. Hence you project onto that person your feelings about the other person that you have known. You relate to the "shadow" rather than to the real person.

The shadow could emerge for different reasons. Sometimes it could be someone's physical appearance, speech, religion, race, role, gender or attitude that results in your experiencing negative feelings. Let us now look at each of these issues.

Personal Psychic Profile 10

YOUR RIGHTS

You do have the right to be heard, but equally you need to listen to others.

You do have the right to assert yourself and so do other people. You do have the right to state what you want, but also you need to recognise others' needs.

You do have the right to feel and realize that other people have emotions, too.

You do have the right to make mistakes and remember that people who never make mistakes, never make anything.

So, avoid playing the game of "Blemish" which is only pointing out their mistakes.

You do have the right to be protected by the law, but also you need to live within the law.

You do have the right to free speech, but remember the effect of your language upon others if you make racist, sexist or abusive comments.

You do have the right to feel secure, but remember that security is a state of mind and comes from within.

You do have the right to be happy, so if you were given a joyless script as a child, then give yourself permission to change it.

You do have the right to be ill, so stop trying to play at martyr.

You do have the right to be treated with respect, but remember, so do others

You do have the right to grieve, so give yourself permission to cry, feel sad and express your feelings.

You do have the right to give others their rights so learn to empower people.

You do have the right to enjoy your sexuality, as long as it is not in the form of harassment or impinges upon others people's boundaries.

You do have the right not to be overlooked, but it is up to you to make your mark and be seen.

You do have the right not to be emotionally abused, however, people cannot read your mind so you need to assertively tell them when you feel this way.

You do have the right not to be physically abused so it is up to you to distance yourself from the perpetrator. This is easier said than done for many people, but if you work on your own feelings of self-worth, then you will reach a stage of recognising that you are no longer prepared to live or work where such behaviour exists.

KEEPING FIT

Well congratulations on finishing the book! I hope you have enjoyed the experience gained from the advice and insights offered. I also hope that you are feeling a lot fitter!

Congratulations on having completed the previous check-up, profile and work out. Now read keeping fit, in order to learn how you have improved. This will help you to create your own fitness pack. It is like having your very own personal trainer. Complete each section so that you have a personal skills awareness and development plan.

As you have discovered, assertiveness is a powerful and empowering skill. But like any skill, practice makes perfect, and the more times you use it, the better you become at that particular skill. Keep practising, keep fit!

Having worked through the book, you now have the opportunity to check out what you have learned.

What do you now think that 'being assertive' means?

	Passive	Assertive	Aggressive
Voice	quiet	clearly audible	loud
Language	Unsure, indirect: maybe, might	Direct and Concise: "I would like, need, have"	Accusative, argumentative: Should, will
Eyes	Lowered	Straight gaze	Glaring or expressionless
Body Language	Withdrawing, retired, hands clasped, lower chin	Upright, shoulders down, open gestures	Pointed finger, curled fists, hands on hips, fingers forward, folded arms and chin forward
Attitudes	"could do better', like to please, easily persuaded, my fault"	"I know what I need and will listen to your needs"	"don't argue with me", think they're right, sexist, stubborn, racist
Feelings	Fear, guilt, inadequacy, unsure, insecure	Confident, self-love, calm, democratic	Anger, frustration, revenge, superior
Early Childhood messages	Turn the other cheek, don't push yourself forward, be nice	As good as anyone else, you're special, you're loved	Stand up for yourself, don't let anyone win, fight, hit back
See Yourself	as inferior	as an equal	as superior

*possible cultural differences

MANAGING CONFLICT SECTION CHECKLIST

Coping with Criticism

What is my preferred way of handling conflict?

> To Avoid
>
> To Appease
>
> To Adapt
>
> To Attack
>
> To Address

What I have learned is that:

_____

I can now:

_____

Dealing with Criticism

When criticised I will say to myself – (insert the correct word)

Is this _____

Or _____

If the criticism is valid I will: _____

If the criticism is invalid I will: _____

When addressing someone about a conflict situation I will be assertive by saying:

"What I have _____

"That makes me _____

"What I _____ is"

EXPRESSING MY VALUES

What are my values that I find difficulty in defending?

_____

To which people in my life am I resistant to state my beliefs and values?

_____

What could happen to me if I did express them?

_____

What is this telling me?

_____

What can I do about this in the future?

_____

Which subjects do I find make me feel:

Angry   _____
Embarrassed   _____
frightened   _____
passionate   _____
judgmental   _____
uncomfortable _____

What language will I use in future?

_____   instead of   _____
_____   instead of   _____
_____   instead of   _____

_____ instead of _____

What specifically could I say in the future to be heard and not overlooked?

_____

Now check out your rights
I now know and believe that I have the following rights. Tick if you agree.
I have the right to have rights
I have the right to be heard
I have the right to assert myself
I have the right to say what you want
I have the right to feel
I have the right to make mistakes
I have the right to be protected by the law
I have the right to free speech
I have the right to feeling secure
I have the right to be happy
I have the right to be ill
I have the right to be treated with respect
I have the right to grieve
I have the right to give others their rights
I have the right to enjoy your sexuality
I have the right not to be overlooked
I have the right not to be emotionally abused
I have the right not to be physically abused

The most important one for me is

_____

The one with which I have the most difficulty doing is

_____

The one that I am really good at is

_____

KEEPING FIT

Well congratulations on finishing this part of the book! I hope you have that you have had at least one 'ah ah' experience. That means when you suddenly recognise, understand or make a connection with a new thought or behaviour. It is one aspect of emotional intelligence when you become more self-aware. Also, I anticipate that you enjoyed the experience gained from the advice and insights offered and I expect that you are feeling a lot fitter!

As you have discovered, assertiveness is a powerful and empowering skill. But like any skill, if you refrain from using it then you become less adapt and lose your edge of fitness. The more times you use it, the better you become at that particular skill. Keep practising, keep fit! This is what the final part of this book is all about.

What do you now think that 'being assertive' means?

Keeping Fit by Accepting and Giving Compliments

You will get so much more out of life if you are able to accept and give compliments. Learn to enjoy, not shrink from, praise. Congratulate people rather than criticize them.

I know you have external pressures and deadlines to meet, but in order to be assertive you need to be relating genuinely to people. Having face-to-face conversations, particularly learning more about your colleagues and managers. So it is vital that you know how to give praise, not in a phoney way, but in a way that builds up and encourages people.

If you experienced lots of praise as a child then you are likely to do this more easily and openly. If, however, you were brought up in a critical environment then you may find that you are behaving in the same way to others.

If you are a parent, sometimes you will recognize yourself saying the same things that were said to you (yes, even things you hated hearing at the time) you just go on re-scripting.

Giving praise may be an important skill for you to practise. You will need to learn to say:

"Well done, I really appreciate that" or

"I thought you did that job really well".

It is essential to recognize that a word of encouragement and appreciation when a job at work or at home, is well done, is better than a tonic for the recipient!

Praise, Praise, Praise!

At work, there is no praise like that of a manager's praise, which if you are one, you will be giving throughout the year. At home, there is no praise like that of your partner or children.

A pat on the back is not very far, anatomically, from a kick in the bottom, but it is a long way psychologically from the resulting different responses.

Keeping Fit – Keeping Your Body Fit by Creating Rapport

Remember that report is spelt RAP ORT.

Sixty to eighty percent of human communication is done non-verbally (Allan Pease 1993).

Yes. In terms of your body language, you are now likely to be aware that certain body positions can trigger certain perceptions in other people's minds. Although you may not really think it matters – wrong! – it does! It is not what messages that you think you are sending, but what is actually being received. Like, "It's not what you say, it's the way that you say it!"

When talking to people with whom you feel comfortable, you are likely to demonstrate this ease by your body gestures. The converse is true.

Next how skilled are you on the ten ways for creating rapport?

Skilled unskilled

1. Smiling ____ ____
2. Keeping warm eye contact ____ ____
3. Being natural, the dance of rapport comes easily. ____ ____
4. Mirroring their body language initially ____ ____
5. Opening up your body position, looking relaxed in order to relax the other person. ____ ____
6. Using appropriate language. ____ ____
7. Adopting voice level and speed in essence with theirs. ____ ____
8. Valuing what is being said, even if you disagree. ____ ____
9. Highlighting what they have said, recognising that it is their true perspective. ____ ____
10. Giving feedback. ____ ____

Consider the following suggestions, and remember, it is not what you think you are communicating, it is what people are seeing and receiving that gets your message across.

If you are assertive then you will gel. If you don't gel then it is likely to be because you are missing a vital ingredient, that is, rapport. If you haven't got rapport you haven't got anything!

Assertive rapport enables you to put people at their ease, gives you an instant insight into how they are feeling, enables you to communicate more effectively, generating a feeling of warmth, even trust. And the good news is that with a little effort on your part you can go a long way towards acquiring this skill!

* Keep as attentive as possible and sit facing the person.
* Readily accepting eye contact.
* Keep your body language open.
* Try to use the same tone or speed of voice when talking with someone.

This can be difficult between genders, but none the less it is possible. If someone is speaking very quickly and you speak very slowly, then there is likely to be little rapport. Also, if they have a high-pitched voice and yours is very low and deep, then there will be little rapport. This is not to say you should mimic the other person, but be aware of slightly modulating your tone and speed as best you can. When people have rapport, often you will hear their voice tones change in essence with each other.

Apart from your voice, there is also the aspect of the language that you use. If you are talking to someone and ask them;

"What do you think about…" and they reply;

"Well, I feel that…" then you are likely to think that they are not answering your question. Equally, if you are asked a question and omit to use their language, then they may think that you don't understand, or you are not on their same wavelength.

A. Ask for what you want.

S. Say, I observe, feel, need.

S. Shift your shadows.

E. Embrace emotions.

R. Realise your rights.

T. Today not tomorrow.

I. Imagining can be worse than reality!

V. Voice your values.

E. Empower yourself with 'no'

Summary

Having worked through the book, you are now likely to be aware of how people's appearance can create all kinds of stereotyping and prejudice. How they dress may affect your feelings towards them. If you are someone who works in a setting where a uniform is part of the culture, then some of this tension is removed, but even so, for some people even a hairstyle could create a source of unease and make you behave in a non-assertive manner.

So, in order to appear assertive, supposedly, wearing a jacket can influence how people will feel towards you and eighty percent of what you say is believed. The theory is, that if you want to look empowered as a woman, then tie back your hair, wear make-up and darker clothes, preferably suits, avoid peep-toed shoes and long earrings as they are considered to be credibility snatchers!

If you want to appear empowered as a man, then wear dark suits, lighter shirt, and socks that match! For both genders, carry a smaller document case rather than a bulging briefcase. Supposedly, you are so organised that you or your secretary have just put into the case the pertinent, relevant papers for your day's work!

Of course, fashions change and what may be an empowering dress code at the beginning of the third millennium, may not be so in another decade.

You may also behave in a non-assertive way because of people's physical appearance, which can be deceptive at the best of times.

Have you ever wanted to ask someone for travel directions and looked around for a suitable person to ask? Then been surprised that be-suited, intelligent looking person was aggressive and lacked clarity, whereas the youth with the scary orange tomahawk hairstyle, dressed in studded leathers was gentle, concise and helpful?

Then there are the moustaches and beards! You may be stereotyping people as aggressive because of their facial hair which looks like the villains you saw in your childhood books, or films and television programmes!

The element of religion is deeply ingrained in many people. So much has been written and discussed about religion, yet it still remains the most explosive of subjects. Therefore, it is hardly surprising that you may have negative feelings towards someone who is of a different religion, if one's early informative years were spent being indoctrinated as to your religious "supremacy". Hence it can create an appeasing or aggressive response in many otherwise assertive individuals.

People from different cultures, different races may create unease in you, again, because of early childhood messages that you were given. It is vital that you become aware of the reasons behind your negativity or fear towards certain people, that is if you really want to be assertive.

Regardless of someone's culture you may still find within any group of people some with whom you relate well and can be assertive and others with whom you find it difficult to assert yourself. Remember that prejudice is built on the fear of the unknown and it is only when you bother to gain knowledge of the person that you can behave in an assertive open honest way.

People's roles can create non-assertive behaviour because of the negative feelings that you experience, in yourself. One reason may be if you think that they do not deserve such a position. Or you may believe that their personality is such that they are unfit to have that particular responsible role, with the attitudes that they hold. Then there is the issue of gender, which again can bring about non-assertive behaviour from both sexes.

It is well documented that more men than women hold managerial positions. Certainly that, in Great Britain, there are significantly whiter than black managers. However, some men and some women will be happy with the imbalance of male to females, whilst others will still feel aggrieved by the situation. Such attitudes can cause people to behave aggressively. Equally, some people feel ill at ease in the company of a particular gender, which leads them to behave in a non-assertive way.

Where do you stand on this issue? As a woman you may think that you have been overlooked for promotion and the job has been given to an inadequate man just because the culture is male dominated and men make the decisions.

Equally, as a man you may think that you have been overlooked for promotion and the job has been given to an inadequate woman just because the current trends are to look for woman managers in order to show how progressive is the organisation. Both situations can lead you to being non-assertive because of feeling cheated or betrayed.

The gender balance of your team or workforce may create negative feelings in you. If you feel more comfortable with one particular gender, then you are likely to be more assertive with them. Your sexual orientation, however, need not necessarily dictate with whom you feel more comfortable working.

It is more likely that there are some women or men to whom you feel negative towards, therefore being non-assertive, not because of their gender, but because of the numerous other reasons that have been discussed.

Then there is the element of your attitudes that can add to your non-assertive behaviour because of feeling negative towards some colleague or individual. If people do not share your attitudes you need to be able to discuss this. Are you able to change your attitudes or are you intolerant of those people who don't change theirs to yours?

How can you change other people's attitudes? In order for you to change attitudes you will need to join them where they are and then bring them over to your viewpoint.

Some theorists reckon that you have to change attitudes before behaviour can change, whilst others argue that if you change people's behaviour then you change their attitudes. Debatable, but what do you believe? Do you try to change people's behaviour or attitudes? Or preferably, both!

Well congratulations on finishing the book. I hope that you have gained from some of the ideas offered to you and with that you are now feeling fitter.

What have you learned about assertive behaviour and what do you need to enhance the rest of your life?

_____

_____

_____

_____

_____

_____

_____

_____

ASSESSMENT 2

Giving and Receiving Compliments (Feedback for Stress)

ACCEPTING AND DISCOUNTING COMPLIMENTS

Being able to give and receive compliments without embarrassment or denial reflects a healthy level of self-worth. How fit are you in giving and receiving compliments?

Look at the scenarios below. Tick your most likely response.

1. Your partner compliments you on your appearance. Is your response likely to be?

    a. I don't feel very attractive.
    b. Thank you. That feels good.
    c. What are you after?

2. Your friend has just met your new partner. How do you respond when they tell you that they think he/she is terrific?

    a. Keep your eyes off! This one's mine!
    b. I doubt if it will last, they'll find someone more interesting than me.
    c. I totally agree with you. We're good together.

3. You are congratulated on your successful results; for example, on an examination; dinner party; driving test; project or sporting event. Which of the following responses are you likely to make?

    a. Thanks! I'm absolutely thrilled with the results.
    b. I should think so; too, after all the hard work, slavery and time I had to put into it.
    c. It was a fluke; call it beginner's luck!

How many times has someone said to you 'I like your hair' and you, with a toss of your hand, pushing it back, have replied 'It needs washing!' Or to 'I like your tie' responded with 'what was wrong with the one that I wore yesterday'. So it is important to be able to assertively accept compliments and not to 'discount' the other person's feelings or thoughts.

The Appeasing response is A, "Thanks but I don't really think it's that good". This response is putting yourself down.

And also inadvertently saying to the other person that they are not a very good judge of quality. In fact, you are discounting their compliment. I t also reflects unhealthy levels of self-worth and self-confidence. having a low self-esteem and also inadvertently saying to the other person that they are not a very good judge of attractiveness.

In fact, you are discounting their compliment.

The aggressive response would be, "What are you after?"

The type of response is suspicious, attacking and hostile.

In question 2–

The assertive response was, "I totally agree with you, we're good together". This is recognising your own worth and celebrating it.

The aggressive response was, "Keep your eyes off, he's mine".

This is demonstrating your defensiveness, possessiveness and jealousy, which are all aggressive attributes.

The passive response was, "They will find someone more interesting".

This is really putting yourself down and you are in danger of evoking the self-fulfilling prophesy of failing into the relationship.

In question 3–

The assertive response would be, "Thanks, I'm absolutely thrilled with the results". This shows that you are able to recognise your achievements.

The aggressive response was, "I should think so too, after all the hard work, slavery and time I've put into it".

This is a resentful reaction to someone, demonstrating an angry and antagonistic attitude.

The passive response would be, "It's a fluke: call it beginner's luck". This shows an inability to believe in your own talent, intelligence, ability and achievement.

GIVING AND RECEIVING COMPLIMENTS

To accept a compliment assertively all you really need to say is "Thank you".

Assertiveness is about having the ability to respect and admit your own self-worth, and that of other people. It is not about behaving in appeasing or aggressive manner, yet it is often confused with these responses.

So, how did you do in the Fitness Assessment?

Question 1

Question 2

Question 3

However, how did you respond in your check up?

QUESTION 1

The assertive response is B, "Thank you. That feels good". This response reflects a healthy level of self-confidence. $\rightarrow$ 5 POINTS.

The Appeasing response is A, "Thanks, but I don't really think it's that good". This kind of passive response is putting yourself down and also inadvertently saying to the other person that they are not a very good judge of quality. In fact you are discounting their compliment. It also reflects unhealthy levels of self-esteem, self-worth and self-confidence. $\rightarrow$ 0 POINTS

The aggressive response is C, "What are you after?" The type of response is suspicious, attacking and hostile. $\rightarrow$ 0 POINTS

SCORE

QUESTION 2

For question 2, the assertive response is C. "Well done, first-rate presentation. I really think it went down well with the client". This is recognizing the worth of your colleague and celebrating it. You are giving him or her well-deserved praise without undermining your own worth. $\rightarrow$ 5 POINTS

The assertive response was, "I totally agree with you, we're good together". This is recognising your own worth and celebrating it.

184

The aggressive response was, "Keep your eyes off, he's mine". This is demonstrating your defensiveness, possessiveness and jealousy, which are all aggressive attributes.

The passive response was, "They will find someone more interesting". This is really putting yourself down and you are in danger of evoking the self-fulfilling prophesy of failing into the relationship.

QUESTION 3

The assertive response would be, "Thanks, I'm absolutely thrilled with the results". This shows that you are able to recognise your achievements.

The aggressive response was, "I should think so too, after all the hard work, slavery and time I've put into it".

This is a resentful reaction to someone, demonstrating an angry and antagonistic attitude.

The passive response would be, "It's a fluke: call it beginner's luck". This shows an inability to believe in your own talent, intelligence, ability and achievement.

Feelings and Emotions

Your job is probably easy! If you did not have your emotions and those of the people around you, with which to deal, it probably would be. So, in order to begin to identify why it is easier for you to be assertive with some people yet not others, please complete the following questionnaire and exercises.

It is better for you to begin by reflecting on what feelings you have towards people before being given the reasons as to why this might be happening. Hence, when you have finished it, then you can turn to evaluate your fitness profile.

WITH WHOM DO YOU WORK WELL?

List the names of five people with whom you work who would fall into one of the two following categories. Try to put five into each column. If you cannot think of five, then it does not matter; simply write down as many as you can.

A: I WORK WELL.   B: DO NOT WORK WELL

—————————————   —————————————
—————————————   —————————————
—————————————   —————————————
—————————————   —————————————

People with whom I find it difficult to state my beliefs

—————————————

—————————————

People that I would really love to be able to tell, what I really think of them

—————————————

—————————————

People that I believe have overlooked my ability

—————————————

—————————————

Keeping Fit and Emotions

In what ways could I change my behaviour in order to feel more at ease in the presence of people that I allow to make me feel

* Nervous
* Put down
* Hurt
* Angry
* Patronised
* Frightened
* Stupid
* Clumsy
* Inadequate
* Devalued
* Untrustworthy

Remember that trust, or a lack of it, is usually a two-way feeling. You cannot expect people to trust you if you don't trust them. Equally, you won't trust them if they don't trust you, so you need to start by trusting other people. It is better to have trusted and had that trust broken, than to go through life distrusting everybody.

Remember, other people do not make us feel these things, we make or let ourselves feel these feelings. Learn that FEELINGS ARE FACTS.

Your job is probably easy! If you did not have your emotions and those of the people around you, with which to deal, it probably would be. So, in order to begin to identify why it is easier for you to be assertive with some people yet not others, please complete the following questionnaire and exercises.

It is better for you to begin by reflecting on what feelings you have towards people before being given the reasons as to why this might be happening. Hence, when you have finished it, then you can turn to evaluate your fitness profile.

SAYING NO

Has any one person appeared frequently?

_____

_____

What is this saying to me?

_____

_____

What stops me from saying No?

_____

_____

What could I gain from saying No?

_____

_____

Do my gains outweigh what stops me?

_____

_____

What can I do about it?

_____

_____

To whom did I find it most difficult to say No?

_____

_____

How could I now behave towards that person?

_____

_____

As you are aware, ancestral voices can prevent you from being assertive by continuing to chat to you. These are messages that you received and imbibed in childhood. They can "hook" you into behaving in non-assertive, manipulative or adaptive ways. They may prevent you from being open and honest and assertive because they present you with unattainable goals, which lower your self-esteem.

Congratulations on having completed the previous check-up, profile and work out. Now read keeping fit, in order to learn how you have improved. This will help you to create your own fitness pack. It is like having your very own personal trainer. Complete each section so that you have a personal skills awareness and development plan.

Interviews are conducted in different manners depending on the level of the job for which you are applying and the recruitment style of the university, college or employer. The two main styles of interviews are:

Type 1: The unstructured interview
This is the normal interview, where candidates are asked questions of a general nature and are expected to respond in a way that they feel appropriate. The final call in terms of suitability of the candidate is often left to the judgement of the interviewers.

Type 2: The structured interview (also called competency-based interview)
Structured interviews are interviews whereby the interviewers have clearly identified the skills required to carry out the job for which you are applying and

are asking specific questions about the skills involved. The questions call for examples of situations in which the candidate has used the relevant skill.

- A typical Type 1 question would be "How do you rate your communication skills and how do you feel they could be improved?"
- A Type 2 question would be along the lines "Describe a situation where you used your communication skills to achieve a particular outcome against all odds"

Generally speaking, recruiters tend to favour Type 1 interviews with a few Type 2 questions thrown in (this is because pure competency-based interviews are very difficult to set up since a thorough analysis of the job is required in order to ascertain which questions would best help select the right candidate).

You will find below a substantial list of questions for both types of interviews. All questions originate from real recent interviews.

TYPE 1 (Unstructured interview) QUESTIONS

- Tell us about yourself
- What made you choose this college/ university/job/career?
- What is your career ambition?
- Where do you see yourself in 3/5/10 years' time?
- Take me through your CV.
- Tell us about your best/worst teacher.
- Tell us about your best/worst classmate.
- What makes a successful student?
- What are your main strengths?
- What areas do you think that you need to work on to improve your ability as a student?
- Give us three adjectives that describe you best.
- What made you choose university/job?
- What do you think will be your biggest challenge here?
- How do you measure success?
- What difficult decisions have you made?
- Do you enjoy studying?
- What would you do in life if money were no concern?

- What concerns you about this job?
- How do you deal with criticism?
- What is the riskiest thing you've ever done?
- What is your approach to resolving conflict?
- Describe an instance where your work was criticised.
- How would you rate your communication skills and what would you do to improve them?
- What type of things makes you angry?
- Do you ever lose your temper?
- Tell me about your hobbies.
- What do you know about us?
- Do you enjoy working?
- What information technology skills do you possess?
- How would you cope with criticism and a complaint against you?
- What was the most important event in your life?

TYPE 2 (Structured interview) QUESTIONS

Organisation & Planning

- Tell me about a time when you set and achieved a goal.
- Tell me about a time when you changed your priorities to meet others' expectations.
- Tell me about a time when you had to change your point of view.

Decision making

- Describe a challenge or opportunity you identified based on your industry knowledge, and how you developed a strategy to respond to it.
- Describe a time you created a strategy to achieve a longer-term objective.
- Describe a time when you used your business knowledge to understand a specific business situation.

Customer focus

- Give an example of how you provided service to a patient/stakeholder beyond their expectations. How did you identify the need? How did you respond?
- Tell me about a time when you had to deal with a patient/stakeholder service issue.
- Describe a situation in which you acted as an advocate within your hospital for your stakeholder's needs, where there was some organisational resistance to be overcome.

Team focus

- Tell us about a situation where you had to bring a difficult person on board and how you went about it.
- Tell me about a situation where your communication skills did not succeed in getting something done?
- Tell me about a time when you worked successfully as a member of a team.
- Describe a situation where you were successful in getting people to work together effectively.
- Describe a situation in which you were a member (not a leader) of a team, and a conflict arose within the team. What did you do?
- Tell me about a time when you coached someone to help them improve their skills or job performance. What did you do?
- Describe a time when you provided feedback to someone about their performance.
- Give me an example of a time when you recognized that a member of your team had a performance difficulty/deficiency. What did you do?
- Describe a recent situation in which you convinced an individual or a group to do something.
- Describe a time when you went through a series of steps to influence an individual or a group on an important issue.
- Give an example of where you've had to work as a member of a multidisciplinary team?

- Describe a situation in which you needed to influence different stakeholders with differing perspectives.
- Tell me about a time when you had to lead a group to achieve an objective.
- Describe a situation where you had to ensure that your "actions spoke louder than your words" to a team.
- Describe a situation where you inspired others to meet a common goal.

27. Managing Conflict

Standing Up for Your Rights

How good are you at standing up for your rights?

You DO HAVE CERTAIN RIGHTS. LAWYERS may disagree with this wording but for the purpose of this book, answer from a moral rather than a legal perspective. Although, I am still aware that again these rights need to be exercised within the law of your own country or culture

Below you have a list of statements. Tick those with which you readily agree and do not have to think about too long.

How good are you at standing up for your rights?

You have certain rights. A solicitor may disagree with this wording but for the purpose of this book, answer from a moral rather than a legal perspective. Although, I am still aware that again these rights need to be exercised within the law of your own country or culture

Below you have a list of statements. Tick those with which you readily agree and do not have to think about too long.

You have the right to have rights
You have the right to be heard
You have the right to assert yourself
You have the right to say what you want
You have the right to feel
You have the right to make mistakes
You have the right to be protected by the law
You have the right to free speech
You have the right to feeling secure
You have the right to be happy
You have the right to be ill

You have the right to be treated with respect

You have the right to grieve

You have the right to give others their rights

You have the right to enjoy your sexuality

You have the right not to be overlooked

You have the right not to be emotionally abused

You have the right not to be physically abused

Addressing Conflict

At Work

If conflict, bullying or sexual comments are not addressed, then;

1. Work productivity is likely to decrease
2. Staff are unhappy if being bullied or harassed
3. A lack of management intervention worsens the situation
4. Ongoing harassment and bullying demotivates people, innovation and energy levels are lowered
5. Time is wasted avoiding the harasser or bully
6. Work time is spent talking about the situation
7. Relationships are jeopardised, probably permanently
8. If trust is once broken it cannot ever be regained to the same extent
9. Work becomes a joyless place to be
10. Ultimately, 'victims' may leave or take legal action against you as a manager or employer

Bullying and sexual harassment are not always overt and many harassers are not necessarily aware of the effects of their behaviour. It can often be through ignorance rather than malice.

The EC Code

Harassment is unacceptable if:

1. Unwanted, unreasonable and offensive to the recipient
2. Use as a basis for employment decisions (e.g. promotion)
3. Creates intimidating, hostile or humiliating work environment

Sexual harassment can be in the form of pestering, annoying, upsetting or wearing someone out with unwanted comments. Language is so important and many people can object to being called 'boy' or 'girl' whilst others may take offence about comments on their physical appearance. Yes, even when they are supposedly meant in fun. You have to be so careful as a manager.

At the other end of the spectrum harassment can be physical abuse against someone's wishes. Other possibilities could include blackmail and rumour mongering which has caused great distress, even suicide, to some people.

10 Managers' Rules – to prevent sexual harassment for men and women

1. Do not turn a blind eye when you have observed inappropriate sexual behaviour
2. Do not tell jokes that may be construed as sexist or offensive
3. Do not collude with sexual stories and rumours about staff – address them
4. Do not refer to a person's sexual anatomy
5. Do not promote anyone with whom you are or were sexually intimate
6. Do not use language that could offend male or female colleagues
7. Do not make homophobic comments
8. Do not touch or embrace staff without their permission
9. Do not promise promotion or job changes in exchange for sexual favours
10. Do not allow posters, calendars etc., of an erotic sexual nature to be displayed

So as a manager you may also have to deal with allegations of bullying or sexual harassment. In these cases you need to be able to deal sensitively with both the accuser and accused. If you do not have a policy you will need to initiate one, below is a checklist for you to consider in terms of understanding and empathising with the person experiencing the harassment. Also a list of suggestions of what you, as a manager may need to do.

The person experiencing harassment needs to:

1. Tell the person that they object to their behaviour or comments.
2. Act as quickly as possible when bullying or harassment occurs.

3. Write down what happened as soon as possible after the event.
4. Be able to say directly how he or she feels and describe the offensive behaviour.
5. Be prepared to tell his/her story in front of the perpetrator.
6. Seek confidential counselling from a trained counsellor.
7. Ask for emotional support.
8. Ask for help in writing the report.
9. Feel able to come into work knowing that he or she is safe from gossip and ridicule.
10. Choose an empathic senior manager who can be trusted to maintain confidentiality.

Managers need to:

1. Be aware that sexuality exists at work.
2. Inform all staff that sexual harassment will not be tolerated in your organisation.
3. Remove offensive posters, calendars etc., displayed in workplaces.
4. Address any comments or behaviour that are observed as sexual harassment.
5. Talk directly to staff about their behaviour if anyone complains.
6. Initially resolve the problem informally but if needed refer to a trained counsellor.
7. Be confidential about what is disclosed to them and ask for a written report of the incidents, if the harassed person is willing.
8. Reassure the harassed person that their future prospects will not be affected by the incident or the allegations (and carry this out).
9. Implement a preventive policy for sexual harassment.
10. Know and understand disciplinary procedures.

So, recognise that your sexuality is likely to affect you and your colleagues at work, both positively and negatively. Positively, because sex can be fun, motivate, excite, relieve stress, enlighten and enhance the workload. Negatively, because it can lead to sexual harassment, jealousy, rejection, betrayal, loss of trust, or job loss.

HEALTH WARNING

Refer staff to a trained counsellor if they need help. This is a specialised skill, which requires training; do not try to do it yourself.

Managing your own sexuality at work

In order to handle your sexuality at work you may wish to consider the following practices and suggestions:

Memories mould motives

Be aware that early sexual messages can influence the way that you and your staff may think, believe and behave.

The fact that the greater percentage of men tend to continue with their early sexual messages would indicate that as a manager you may think about asking some of your staff what their early messages were and if they continue to carry such thoughts. Do not be surprised if some of them say 'sex was never discussed as a child' but now 'I talk about sex very easily'. It could be that they will jest but not necessarily feel comfortable discussing issues that are about differing gender roles from what they have been brought up to believe; or they may be averse to the appointment of gay candidates; or for the men or women they might find it difficult working with a woman as their line manager. Look out for statements made to you in private about their real beliefs and values in such matters.

Permanent prejudices

Take account of the way in which your early messages (maybe even those about race, religion, sexual orientation or gender) have left you with in-built prejudices and stereotyping.

These actually may affect you in discussion on sexual issues such as forming policies on HIV, establishing medical services for contraception or abortion referrals, initiating or finding accommodation for gay groups, crèches or taking affirmative action when making appointments to positions of power so that women, all races, disabled people or people of a different sexual orientation to yourself are represented.

Courting conflict

Realise that your early sexual messages can be changed but if not, remind yourself that, as a male manager, it is possible that you may be experiencing inner conflict about your sexuality.

As a female manager, remember that many male colleagues maybe undergoing inner conflict, with you as a woman line manager. This could also be the case for many of your staff for whom you have managerial responsibilities. Maybe you can think of someone you know that could be struggling with their job role because of the person with whom they have to work.

Meetings can marginalize

Try to analyse the sexual dynamics in meetings. If you are a lone woman or man surrounded by colleagues all of the same sex, then you may feel isolated or marginalised. On the other hand you may enjoy the scenario. If so, ask yourself why.

Some women, or men, may prefer to be the only woman or man in a management team. It gives them that extra knowledge about their gender and some may even enjoy 'the Thatcher position' as a woman but actually work at preventing other women from joining them, rather than encouraging female promotions. Statements like 'I am the only woman on the executive' can be heard as 'I made it other women can't'. It is a proud comment rather than a sad one.

Lovers liaisons break loyalty

Acknowledge that staff may feel negative emotions about the issue of confidentiality, if you or other managers are involved in 'pillow talk' or a sexual liaison with their colleagues. This can certainly lead to conflict.

Imagine that you have a line manager that is sexually involved with someone for whom you have a line management responsibility. You are dissatisfied with that member of staff's work. You want to discuss it with your line manager but you can't because you know that he or she will have discussed your managerial incompetence or mistakes with their lover (your line manager). It does not make for an easy life and can create a lot of conflict. Sometimes you may be circumvented and decisions arrived at between the two of them in private may not be what you would wish. Cases have been illustrated where staff only have access to the director through their mistress, wife, lover or husband. This certainly creates annoyance, frustration even anger amongst staff. If couples are openly a problem then you as a manager have to establish a management structure that splits up such couplings so that other staff are able to work effectively and not be blocked by such strong twosomes.

Organise your organisation
Sexual stories

Sensitise yourself to your organisation's sexual messages and stories and ask yourself if you may well be contributing towards them. What sexual messages do you emit?

Are you demonstrating a liaison with someone, are you talked about because of your present or past sexual involvements with colleagues? Maybe you have confided in another member of staff about your liaison and that confidence has been broken, so now rumours have whizzed around the workplace. Maybe the relationship has broken down and the aggrieved partner has had their say about your shortcomings. If you hear stories about other people do not add to the rumour. If you are going to say anything then speak to the people concerned.

Preventive policies

Introduce policies that are clear and concise and acceptable to staff, that declare openly the reasons for separating staff into different working areas or roles, especially in cases where particular liaisons are affecting others.

If you are told by someone that they are having problems because of a particular liaison then you need to address the situation. Only talk about what you have observed to them, not what other people have said to you. Say 'What I have observed is that you and ... are now seen as an item and this appears to be causing problems' as two of the staff do not appear to be working effectively in your team. It seems to me that they no longer have direct access to you as their line manager. That makes me feel concerned because previously you all operated well together. What I need is for you to resolve this situation by talking to the members of your team and establishing some ground rules. Ask them if there are any issues that they want to discuss with you, in the presence of your partner. If you say that you have observed rather than what you have been told, you will be listened to. People feel threatened if they think other staff have been telling you tales. If you say what you feel, people cannot argue with how you feel, they can argue with how you think but they cannot say 'you don't feel that'. Be clear in your own mind what you need from your staff. Prepare what you are going to say, don't just waffle then say it directly.

Handling harassment

Deal with issues of sexual harassment, at first in a confidential way, and be sure of your facts and procedures. Avoid projecting your values and belief systems on to others.

Try to remain as objective as possible as sexual harassment often involves an imbalance of power. That is to say that usually it is the harasser who has the power which means that the harassed can have great difficulty in complaining to the powers that be about someone in their power band. You may think that sexual harassment is about lust for the other person but harassment is more likely to be about wanting power over someone and in fact a dislike rather than a fondness for that individual.

Potent power

Think about power issues, how some managers in your organisation use their sexual or gender power over others (for instance if one gender is under-represented).

Some people are also sexually excited by power and maybe some of your staff or customers will be investing power in you. As a manager you will need to be able to distinguish when you are being propositioned because of your position and influence. Some staff may see you as a step on the promotion ladder if they endear themselves to you at whatever level of intimacy, regardless of your gender or sexual orientation. Also be aware of staff who may either threaten to accuse you of harassment because of your position. Or, regardless of your power, truly feel that you are harassing them. So you need to guard yourself against such accusations therefore it is important that you use inoffensive language and relate openly and genuinely to your staff as against in a sarcastic, sniggering, or slimy manner. Other power issues may be seen in the fact that you have the power or influence to appoint your paramours to positions of power. Be warned, this will really cause angst.

Different desire drives

Empathise with staff who are of a different sexual orientation to yourself.

Within your organisation you will be working with people who do not share your particular sexual orientation just as you will be working with people of a different race, culture, religion, gender, all of which needs to be recognised. Prejudice is built on fear and ignorance. So you will need to manage your own fears and ignorance. Try to see the world through their eyes, listen through their ears, walk in their shoes. Sly comments can hurt even the most outwardly successful manager or employee. If you are heterosexual then remember that many homosexuals are scared of revealing their gay orientation for fear of the prejudice that they may have to endure at work. If you are homosexual then try to remember that heterosexuals may only see the world as having one type of sexual coupling so can often make assumptions in their speech and behaviour. This would also apply to the hurt that can be caused by assuming people have partners or families. Peoples' stories are different but their hurt feelings are the same.

Right roles

Recall that your perceptions of sex roles and sex stereotyping may not be shared by others and that different generations may have different attitudes.

Depending upon your age, maybe you have a generation gap with some of your colleagues about sexual stereotyping. Forgetting political correctness for the moment say out loud (unless you are reading this with others present) what you really honestly think the role of a man should be. Is what you have said very different from what you would say at a management meeting? Now try the same thing with what you truly think the role of a woman should be! Again any contradictions between what you say at work and what you inwardly feel? Certain generations grow up with different male and female role models so there are many older managers who still find it difficult to accept the changing role of men and women as we move to the next millennium. However, regardless of age, some men and women are still chauvinistic about their gender and find it difficult to work with the opposite sex in any kind of respecting or genuine way. To work in this negative way can only bring you misery either in a joyless relationship or organisation. Of course, there are many reasons why you might not work well with certain individuals regardless of their gender. They may have 'shadows' – this means that they may remind you of people you have known in the past to whom you attribute negative or positive sexual or emotional feelings.

Curtail conflict

Address issues of conflict with staff when sexual incidents have been reported to you.

Try using phrases like 'What I have observed … That makes me feel … What I need is …' This is mentioned in how to deal with sexual liaisons between colleagues but it is also important to use this approach if you are dealing with the conflict of sexual incidents being reported to you. Get people to say exactly what they have seen not what they have heard rumoured or reported. Ask them how they feel not what they think and do not accept 'I feel that you should do something about it' – that is not a feeling that is a thought. 'I feel frustrated (unhappy, angry, anxious, frightened, hurt, scared, put down or embarrassed etc.) by their behaviour' would be a feeling. Then ask them what they need – 'I need them to be more professional'. This won't do – it is too woolly, get them to be specific. 'I need them to work in different offices'. Then you have to have the skills to address the person who is creating the conflict because of a certain sexual incident. 'I have observed that you touch Susan's bottom when you are working at the desk. That makes me feel anxious. I need you to stop it'. You may want to talk about messages being misconstrued or suggest that Susan is consulted about the complaint but it is important to be direct and precise as illustrated and not beat about the bush. Although the example is of addressing a man it could equally apply to a woman who you consider to be acting inappropriately.

Investigative interviews

In order to avoid unnecessary upsets amongst your staff which can demotivate and even end in industrial tribunals it is essential that your interviews are absolutely fair. If staff complain and consider that people have been appointed or promoted because of their sexual involvement with certain personnel then interviews will have to be investigated. So it is vital that proper procedures are followed not only because of sexual involvement's or liaisons but in all cases. As Baroness Blackstone, Education Minister endorsed in Face the Facts (September 1997). She was interviewed about the complaints received about a chief executive who appointed his mistress as his personal assistant, They later married and then she was promoted to head of personnel. According to the staff interviewed this meant that any complaints or criticisms of him had to be channelled through his wife. The Baroness responded by saying that she was unfamiliar with the with the details of the case but in these situations the interviews would need to be retrospectively investigated. She commented that:

- the procedure must comply with the law
- the job would have to be advertised
- the element of competition needs to be assessed
- a proper interview board must be set up
- the partner should not take part in the interview

So, remember that when there are conflicts of interest and known or emotional associations then you have to be above reproach in any inquiry or investigation into the interview.

Summary

So, in terms of your organisation, it is vital that you have guidelines of acceptable and non-acceptable behaviour. If you haven't got these then set up policies for 'sex' or 'love' at work. Establish an understanding and a formula with your staff about how they can complain if certain sexual relationships are affecting them or others at work.

Whilst in terms of managing your own sexuality:

- Remember that it is natural to have sexual feelings, but they may take up a lot of your 'psychic energy'.
- Check out your feelings, if you feel uncomfortable in someone's presence it may be that they have a 'shadow' of someone you know or it may be because you are sexually attracted to them.
- Explore your attitudes towards sexuality and individuals. You may be attracted to someone but recognise the consequences of your becoming sexually involved with someone at work.
- Question your sexual feelings and the emotions that you may have towards other colleagues or customers and ask yourself if these feelings are affecting your decision making or working life.
- Treat yourself to further training on how to handle sexual issues at work
- Enjoy your sexuality. It is a vital element of your being.

Coping with Conflict

Conflict happens because everyone is different. We have:

- Different needs
- Different perceptions
- Different expectations

Conflict can be positive. Some of the differences between people can lead to change. This is how people develop new attitudes, successful collaborations and new solutions to problems, both at home and at work. But conflict can be negative, especially when it is not dealt with, leading to unhappiness and even physical illness.

People deal with conflict in different ways and understanding these styles of interaction can help.

Different Types of Conflict

First of all consider the different types of conflict that people experience.

1. *Inner Conflict:*

When you are being pulled in opposite directions. You may have inner conflict between home and work. What you want to do as opposed to what you have to do. You may have conflict between your belief system and what is expected of you as an employee, partner or parent.

2. *Conflict between you and one other person:*

When you have to say something to someone. Something they do upsets you. Maybe you don't have the necessary skills or confidence to address the situation, but this is likely to be the type of conflict that you will need to know how to handle.

3. Conflict between two people:

For whom you have some responsibility. This maybe your colleagues, employees, or your children. You may have to manage and resolve it.

4. Team/Family conflict:

When someone in a group is behaving in a way that is negatively affecting other members of that working group.

Different Ways of Handling Conflict

There are five ways of dealing with hostility or violence. Which option would you choose in the following situation?

A customer complains to you about their anger at the bureaucratic system that has prevented them from being fairly treated. What do you do?

1. Agree with them about the stupid rules.
2. Tell them they deserve it and that it appears that it is their fault?
3. Ask them to tell you the facts of the case and act on the evidence presented.
4. Say, "It's nothing to do with me".
5. Say "Don't worry, it will turn out all right".

So the five ways are

AVOIDING	(answer d)
APPEASING	(answer e)
ATTACKING	(answer b)
ADAPTING	(answer a)
ADDRESSING	(answer c)

Which one did you choose? People's styles depend on how important goals and relationships are to them. Ideally, you need to aim to ADDRESS conflict.

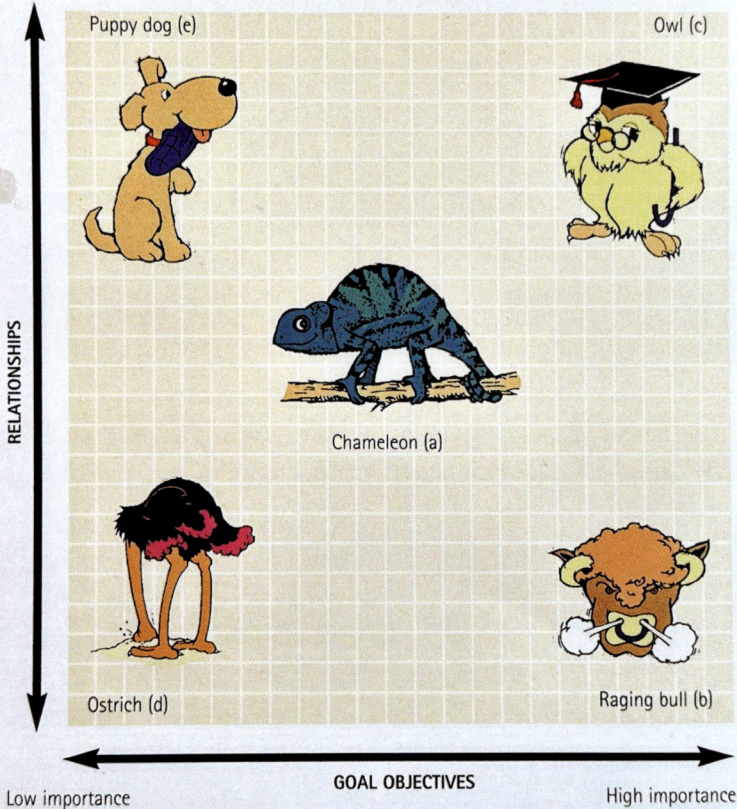

High importance

Puppy dog (e)   Owl (c)

RELATIONSHIPS

Chameleon (a)

Ostrich (d)   Raging bull (b)

GOAL OBJECTIVES

Low importance   High importance

THERE ARE FIVE WAYS OF HANDLING CONFLICT...

ADAPTING (a), **ATTACKING** (b), **ADDRESSING** (c), **AVOIDING** (d), **APPEASING** (e).

Which one did you choose?

People's styles depend on how important goals and relationships are to them.

Ideally, you need to aim to **ADDRESS** conflict.

How Do YOU Handle Conflict?

Begin by answering the following questions:

1. Do you dislike conflict or violence?   Yes____ No____

2. List five words that describe conflict.

    _____

    _____

3. What feelings do you associate with conflict?

    _____

    _____

4. With whom are you most likely to come into conflict?
    (List their real or anonymous names)

    _____

    _____

5. What are the three most likely situations that cause conflict, violence or
    aggressiveness for you?

    _____

    _____

    _____

6. If you have no conflicts (or very few) what may you deduce about:

a. Yourself

    _____

b. The staff with whom you work

    _____

c. Your relationships with people?

    _____

7. How do you tend to resolve conflict?

	YES	NO
By my people skills		
By negotiating with the person		
By saying what I need		
By talking to others about the situation		
By looking for another job		
By compromising		
By grumbling to others		
By avoiding issues		
By attacking others		
By being pleasant to other people		
By addressing the situation		

8. Complete the following statement by ticking the appropriate box: "When I address conflict, generally…"

	YES	NO
I lose	____	____
I win	____	____
Neither of us wins	____	____
We both win	____	____

9. The reason for the former is because I

_____

10. When I do try to resolve difficult issues with another person, the skills I use are

_____

Helpful Tips

Positive thinking – I'm OK you're OK

If you are *imagining* the worst thing that can happen, your body will respond accordingly. Maybe you will begin to sweat, or your heart will beat faster, or your guts will begin to churn. If you think positively you can avoid this.

Start from the psychological state of thinking that you are OK and that the other person is OK. Empower yourself, rather than investing power in the other person, regardless of their status or reputation. Everyone is equal, in terms of his or her emotions. Virtually all people feel happy when valued and rejected when critically dismissed.

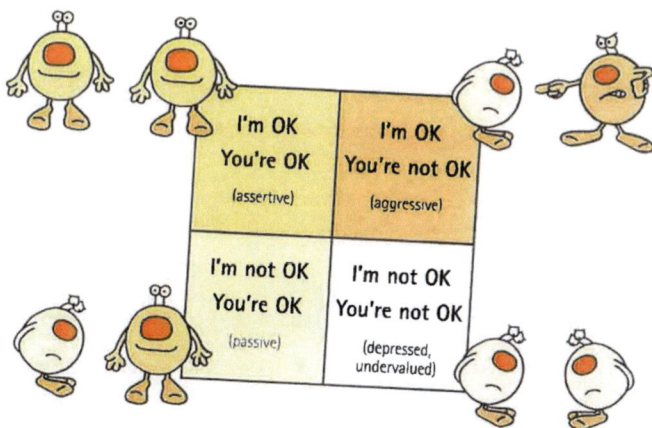

I'm OK You're OK (assertive)	I'm OK You're not OK (aggressive)
I'm not OK You're OK (passive)	I'm not OK You're not OK (depressed, undervalued)

Body Language

Remember, you communicate with 7% of your words. 38% with your voice and 55% with your body language.

Avoid

- pointing your finger;
- clenching your fists;
- putting your hands on your hips;
- "steepling" your hands;
- putting your arms behind your head;

- fiddling with hair, beard or glasses;
- turning up your foot;

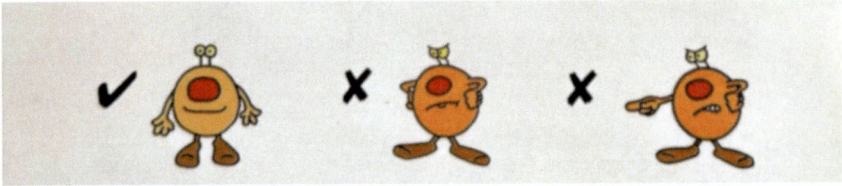

Any of the above postures and traits show signs of your uncomfortableness.

Therefore, you may need to sit, or stand, in an uncomfortable position for you, in order to be perceived as being in control and or ready to resolve any issue or concern.

In potentially violent situations

Avoid changing your movements quickly from the norm. Like jerky movements from smooth or vice versa.

Avoid making agitated movements.

Creating Rapport

- Face the person.
- Stand, or sit, in an open posture;
- Keep arms and legs uncrossed;
- Mirror their body language;
- Reflectively, hold your head at the same angle as theirs;

In order to create rapport you may have to 'Fake it, till you make it.' When you are feeling anxious or uncomfortable in the presence of someone, by placing your body in positive positions, you will become more confident.

Active Listening

That means listen with your ears, eyes, heart and brain. Listen to the music behind the words!

Reflecting What You Have Heard

By reflecting (repeating out loud) what you think is the issue or the concern, you are then able to let the other person know that you have listened and they can then tell you if they think that you have understood or misunderstood what they have said.

Language

When addressing someone, about their behaviour or attitude, then use specific language and get to the point quickly.

First say "What I have observed is…"
Then say "That makes me feel…"
Followed by "What I need is…"

By saying, "What I have OBSERVED", you avoid being questioned on "who told you?" and the person feels less threatened. By disclosing your feelings, no one can argue with how you FEEL but they can argue with how you THINK. They cannot say, "You don't feel angry" or whichever feeling is present.

Be honest about your feelings. Expressing feelings is not a sign of weakness, but a sign of strength. It takes a very secure person to disclose their feelings. By stating what you NEED you let the person know where they stand, what they have to do, how they have to behave, and what is acceptable and what is inappropriate. Too often, people go all around the houses trying to get to the point but omit to state their actual needs.

Selecting Your Words

Your speech might include using certain words that create a feeling of unease in yourself or others. Or certain words will affect how your customers and colleagues or family and friends relate to you.

Try to use:	Instead of:
working *with*	Working *for*
address	confront or tackle
issues or concerns	problems
could	Ought or should
What happened to make you late?	Why were you late?

211

Voice

As well as the words themselves, there is the way in which you speak. Many people still have misconceptions about the difference between an aggressive and assertive voice and language. So you may be using the right words, but speaking in an abrupt, chipped way. Certain accents and dialects may irritate you. Yours' may irritate others. You cannot do much about that, but at least be aware that you may be dismissing someone just because of the way they speak.

Being Tolerant

Just how tolerant are you in terms of recognizing that people have different values from you and often-different expectations of you. Your perceptions of an individual's behaviour, or what they are trying to say to you, can be very different from theirs'. Attempt to be tolerant of others perceptions of their world.

Then there is the element of attitudes that can add to your feelings of hostility or your even creating aggressiveness in others. If people do not share your attitudes you need to be able to discuss this. Are you able to change your attitudes or are you intolerant of those people who don't change theirs to yours?

In order for you to change attitudes you will need to join them at where they are and then bring them over to your viewpoint.

Some theorists reckon that you have to change attitudes before behaviour can change, whilst others argue that if you change people's behaviour then you change their attitudes. Debatable, but what do you believe? Do you try to change people's behaviour or attitudes? Maybe both.

Your own attitude to others is vital. If you are positive towards them then they are more likely to respond positively towards you, and the reverse is true.

What is your attitude regarding loyalty to your colleagues? Do you have team loyalty? Or do you talk about them behind their backs, when you have some conflict issue with which to deal, in the hope that you can influence other people's attitudes towards them or you? Loyalty has to be earned both ways.

So maybe you should start by talking *to* people, not *about* them.

28. Handling Criticism

Almost all of us are criticised from time to time.

Think of it as 'feedback with love' it may make you feel better. When it is appropriate, I always head my 'feedback with love' as I mean it. I am not trying to put the person down, upset them, criticise them as a human being with feelings, but to say cleanly and honestly what I am thinking or feeling about our communication. Just what is the point in your being dishonest, smarmy, two faced, sycophantic in your behaviour?

Firstly

1. **Listen to the criticism carefully**, rather than rejecting it or arguing with the person. For many people their first response is usually to justify their behaviour or decisions.
2. **Ask yourself whether the criticism is VALID or INVALID** and/or whether it FEELS it is in the form of a put-down.

If the criticism is VALID:

   a. Acknowledge that it is true, **say sorry**. If someone is delighting in 'having a go' at you, saying sorry is one way of 'knocking them off balance.'
   b. When the criticism is generalised, then ask for more information.

3. **Ask for the critic to be more specific with actual examples.**

   a. If several are involved, then check out with others ask them as to whether or not they also experiencing you in a similar way.
   b. Decide whether or not you are going to change your behaviour as a consequence of the criticism.

c.   Thank the critic for giving you their feedback.

Secondly

If the criticism is INVALID:
Say so and explain calmly your reasons for the situation being discussed.

1.   If the criticism is valid but in the form of a put-down:

Acknowledge that YES, the criticism is true. However, address the put-down and say how you feel about how the person is behaving towards you or the language that they are using.

2.   If the criticism is INVALID but in the form of a put-down

Say 'that is not true'. Address the put-down and say how it makes you feel. People cannot argue with how you feel. So, say –

'What I have observed … That makes me feel … and What I need is … and remember 'We all have our own truth.'

There will be times when you are criticized, so it is important that you are able to handle criticism in a way that is productive to both you and the critic.

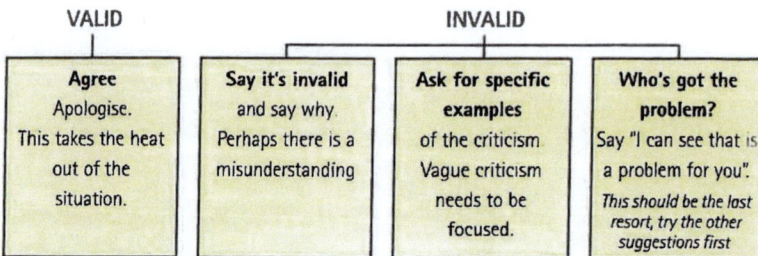

VALID	INVALID		
Agree Apologise. This takes the heat out of the situation.	**Say it's invalid** and say why. Perhaps there is a misunderstanding	**Ask for specific** **examples** of the criticism. Vague criticism needs to be focused.	**Who's got the** **problem?** Say "I can see that is a problem for you". *This should be the last* *resort, try the other* *suggestions first*

EXERCISE 1

Think of an example when someone has criticized you:

1. What exactly did they say?
2. How did you respond?
3. What was the outcome?
4. Now ask yourself:
5. Was the criticism valid or invalid?
6. If it was valid criticism, did you agree with them?
7. If it was invalid criticism, did you disagree with what the person said and say why it was invalid?
8. Was the criticism vague?
9. Did you ask them to give you specific examples of their criticism of your behaviour?
10. Who had the problem?
11. What could you do differently next time?

How Do You React to Criticism?

Some people start to justify their behaviour while others say nothing but feel angry or upset. Others respond by blaming someone else. How do you react?

First of all you will need to decide if the criticism is valid or invalid.

VALID	INVALID		
You never meet deadlines	Say it's invalid	Ask for specific examples	Who's got the problem?
Yes? Then agree			

Giving Feedback

As well as receiving criticism you may have to criticise others.

- Be specific; give instances rather than being vague.
- Comment on **behaviour** that can be changed, rather than on the person himself or herself.

- Recognize that *you* may be wrong and that the other person could have a good and valid reason for what has happened; you will not know about it unless you ask them.
- Recognize your prejudices and stereotyping.

Violence, aggression or hostility can be exacerbated if someone perceives you as being prejudiced. Sometimes you may be prejudiced (another word? – 'feel an instinctive dislike?') against someone because of their physical appearance, their race, culture, religion, and geographical place of birth, even their name. Whatever the reasons, you need to be able to deal with them in a rational way. Try to think of people as equals with the same emotions as yourself.

If you are no nearer understanding why you feel negative towards certain customers or individuals, then consider if the idea of "shadowing" helps. You may be working with someone and experiencing a sense of feeling uncomfortable, you are not sure why you feel like this, as they have not directly upset you. This could because the person reminds you of someone else that you have known before, that created negative feelings in you.

Bullying

Bullying can range from having rumours spread about you to being made to do something that is illegal. You may be constantly criticized, threatened, humiliated, embarrassed, denied information, or support. You may even be being called names, teased, pawed, hit, attacked, ignored, or told that you are stupid.

Bullies are usually insecure people who have severe, personal problems. They will target anyone who is vulnerable, maybe they are physically ill or having family or work problems. Bullies do not target people who are successful, happy and well-liked by others.

Try to remember that THE TRUTH HURTS. Recognize that when someone says something to you that hurts you it is probably because you believe it about yourself. If they say something that doesn't hurt then it is likely that you don't believe it.

If it hurts ask yourself "do I believe this about myself?" If you do then try to identify who first started to say such things about you. Are you still living that 'script'? You don't have to you can change it. Think ' I am not here to live up to your expectations of me nor are you here to live up to my expectations of you.'

Name calling

Hurts	Doesn't hurt
I believe it	I do not believe it
Why? Who first made that comment about me?	Try saying 'sounds like you are talking about yourself'

Feeling Bullied?

Do you think that you have conflict because you are being bullied? If so then it is important that you talk to the person concerned. For instance, 'I do not like you speaking to me in that way. I feel insulted and need you to stop using that phrase.' If the bullying persists then tell someone, preferably your line manager, about the bullying. Workplaces are required to take note of unacceptable behaviour.

Sexual Conflict at Work

Sexual feelings happen at work just as much as anywhere else, but sometimes these feelings may badly affect working relationships. Other staff may have difficulties with sexuality between their colleagues. Harassment should not be tolerated and most workplaces now have a sexual harassment policy. Like bullying, it may help to share your concerns with others.

If you have to deal with sexual harassment make sure all disclosures are treated in confidence. Listen with empathy to staff's concerns about sexual behaviour at work. Try to remember that sexuality is a basic drive. It is ok to feel sexual but it is not ok to offend others with your needs. Keep an open mind when discussing items of a sexual nature, everyone has their own truth. People will change their history in order to deal with the present. Watch your language to prevent offence. Organize a policy that covers relationships at work and keep a record of complaints about sexual issues

Jeanie Civil MSc psych
August 2001

29. What Kind of Animal Are You?

Remember this earlier, now reflect on it, any changes you think you may make or have already made? Are you an owl yet?

30. Motivation

What Motivates You?

It is often a difficult thing to know about yourself. Are you searching for love, approval, money, recognition, power, influence, personal gratification of a hobby, project, respect, justice, status, a better life for your children, status, saving the planet, a belief in your God, proving that your teachers, or others were wrong when they said that you would never make anything of yourself, or being told that you were a failure in something ? Or maybe being more successful than your siblings, a better house or garden, or trying to forget abuse, or the death of a parent as a child or giving your children the opportunity that you never had, or trying to find a relationship by where you will not be rejected again, or are you motivated to try to love yourself despite your personal story?

Think back, how are you feeling, what kind of behaviour are you recalling about yourself?

Motivation involves the biological, emotional, social, and cognitive forces that activate our behaviour. Wow that is a mouthful. In everyday psychology motivation describes why a person does something. What are our needs, what drives us, activates us and how do we direct ourselves to achieve our goals or dreams?

Have you ever thought why am I doing this? I did, when producing the village pantos, mainly because friends said why do you do it, it takes up so much of your time? After a long time, I decided that one of the motivators for me was that I just love working with kids, it takes me back to the time in my life as a nursery nurse when life held so much opportunity, hope and dreams for me. It is being with kids that offers me an honest clean relationship, that is game free, so genuine and the openness and belief that they invest and give me.

"So, what motivates you in your life?"

Most people have no idea why they want to wake up each morning (apart from they don't want to die) or what they want to do with their life.

Ordinary people wake up each morning because they have to go to work. And the reason they go to work is that they want to get paid. They want to pay their bills and expenses. In other words, they are working for the money. However, their motivator as to what they do with the money may be to look after their family or to give to charities or to show off by having that expensive envious holiday?

Why do you do what you do in your life? You do something because you want to gain pleasure or to avoid pain. This is why people who do not need to work for money or when they do not have go to work, they choose not to work, probably sleep later but still try to avoid pain and to gain pleasure. Maybe they still want to work voluntarily because that brings them the feeling of being needed and valued. Or perhaps you feel pleasurable now reading this. Everything we do, **we do because of these two forces, pain and pleasure**.

Most people who are motivated by money, think that what they want in life is money and having the next shiny objects, but what they never realised is that the physical things that they want are just the means to an end. What they are truly searching after is the **feeling** of owning the items. If you are chasing money for the reward – is it the money? Or is it for the feeling? What life feeling are you searching for, I guess mine is love?

Other major motivators are the *Desire to be The Best.* While some people are motivated by *Helping others.* They want to see changes in people's lives and they want to fight for a better future for the world. While not everyone is driven to help others, but if you are, it is good. You achieve the 'helpers high'. There is another group of people who are motivated by *Power and fame.* Politicians are a great example here. Others are inspired to become the leader and they are driven to achieve greater power and fame in life. Sometimes experienced as control freaks. *Recognition* is another factor that makes certain people motivated. They want to prove that either they are right or someone is wrong. The final factor that motivates most people in their lives is *Passion.*

Why do you think some people do what they do? Why do you think they are willing to wake up early and work harder than others? The answer is that they are passionate about what they do. Think about it, are there times when you feel so motivated for something that you are willing to wake up early, sacrifice your sleep and leisure time for it. This is why passion is important because it can drive you each day to achieve what you want in life. Sadly, most people never develop their passion in their work. They work like a zombie without feeling any passion.

They make sure they are not the first one to reach the office and not the last one to leave.

Think about what your mind is recalling and what it is telling you about yourself, how is that making you feel and what behaviour may you change in the future to be happier, at peace with yourself and mentally well?

31. Setting Goals

After Covid many people will be setting themselves new goals right now, are you?

Goal setting is the first step we make towards planning for the future.

With so much unemployment and people trying to set new goals for their future employment, so many parents and children anxious about returning to school, having to set new goals for child care arrangements, many adults, both young and old, anxious about their health risks as they try to set themselves may be too many goals too quickly in order to try and achieve a more interactive social life; the lack of financial security and the fear of losing their present-day homes and lifestyle and also for the thousands of people who will be grieving over the loss of their loved ones.

A psychological definition for goal setting refers to a successful plan of action that we set for ourselves.

You will probably have heard of setting SMART goals. This acronym stands for: Specific, Measurable, Attainable, Relevant and Time-bound.

So, when setting yourself goals you need to be Specific about what it is exactly that you want to achieve; how will you Measure the goal to know if you have achieved it? Ask yourself if the goal is Attainable or are you pushing yourself too far? Is it Relevant to what you want to achieve or how you want to feel?

Have you ever heard anyone say 'some time, someone, will do something about this?' Yes, that is why so many things never get done because nobody is specifically named to achieve or do a particular task by a given time. Particularly at meetings. It needs to be decided who, what and by when?

The Benefits of Goal Setting

- Provides **Direction**. First and foremost, goals give you a **direction** and destination … Clearer focus on what is important …

- Clarity in decision making ...
- Gives you control of your future ...
- Provides motivation ...
- Gives you a sense of personal satisfaction ...
- Gives you a sense of purpose in life ...

Changing habits as well as goal setting are very beneficial for your mental health

So, tips for setting goals are:

- Set Clear, Specific and Realistic Goals ...
- Take small steps not giant leaps ...
- Get support ...
- Share your goals with others ...
- Stay positive ...
- Celebrate your successes and challenges ...

What future goals are you setting for yourself right now for the coming few months?

32. Meetings

ZOOM. What? No not Zoom. Zoom for me was a word learned in my childhood from my comic's days – Zoom Bang Wallop. Many older people will remember them I am sure.

Psychologists would and do, notice many personality traits in all meetings coming to the fore, perhaps because of the power it offers some of telling you what to do, putting you into rooms, excelling in their controlling behaviour in the meetings but here we are now with so many new skills that we have been learned during Covid 19.

Whilst zoom meetings have had their plus points, usually quicker time-wise, avoids time-wasting travel and certainly offers certain personalities the chance to excel in their controlling behaviour, that may or may not be received favourably by many onlookers. So, this is nothing to do with those Zoom meetings that many have disliked, whilst others have thoroughly enjoyed them. However, they do not offer us the importance of the vital skills we need to use in face to face meetings.

Meetings; Feel Before They Think.

Maybe you have attended meetings where you have picked up the awkwardness in the room or the embarrassing silence. Ones that you have gone to when you feel that you are not really wanted, more there by title than what you really ever contribute.

Is this to do with the subject or the people with whom you are expected to value and respect, when you don't? Anyway this is about the psychology that happens in meetings when you can see people's reactions, hear the tone of their voice, watch their body language, read the group, make eye contact, notice the looks that are passed between people who are laughing, sneering or just plainly bored by the present speaker.

Process and product

Product-prepare and read the minutes and note anything that you may want to enquire about. If you set the agenda give a name who is leading the discussion and a time indicator. Guess you know those tricks of putting controversial items at the end of the meeting when people vote for anything to finish and leave.

Process

Feelings can be heated and passionate people may be unable or unwilling to be a 'yes' person as also will many never say anything because they do not want to look stupid or are worried about losing face or just hate conflict so never address it.

Hidden agendas are around in all meetings. What do you remember in your last meeting anyone trying to impress or looking for approval or patronising?

Some want to get their own way having rallied support outside the meeting some people who you may not like and you just close your ears when they start one day, they may just say something worth listening to.

When you see two people whispering to each other in your proximity, the paranoid side of you comes out. Don't assume they're criticising you or plotting your demise. Just say one meeting at a time please. Or would you like to share that?

Avoid letting any one person dominate the discussion. People will often speak out of turn for their own self-validation. If you notice this, quickly direct the discussion elsewhere. If someone isn't speaking out or contributing, direct a question their way or ask them what they think or how they feel about a certain idea.

It's vital to uphold good morale throughout the meeting – If there is any bad news, it's best to open with it and get it out of the way quickly. Try to keep things positive and avoid any negative discussions. Jokes can lighten a mood.

There's usually a lot more going on in a meeting than what is actually being said. The psychology of meetings includes certain body language give a ways, folded arms, upturned feet – a sign of being uncomfortable with what they are saying or what is being asked of them, reactions to certain topics, and even the seating arrangement. Watch out for anyone sitting opposite the chair, sign they are vying for their job or influence. Of course, it could be the last seat left when you arrive. Posture and fidgeting during are often indicators of unease, boredom, or frustration. Yawning – boredom overcome with tiredness.

Some people always have to say something whilst others only speak when they have something to say.

So which meetings do you like to attend (if any) and which ones are you glad when they are over?

33. What Is Said...May not Be What Is in the Mind

At the meeting what they are really thinking. At the meeting and what is thought. Spot the difference.

_____

_____

In meetings, many aspects of an agenda are covered and almost everybody voices an opinion at some point, however there are hidden agendas. Many statements are delivered and openly made, however what is spoken may not be what their mind is thinking?

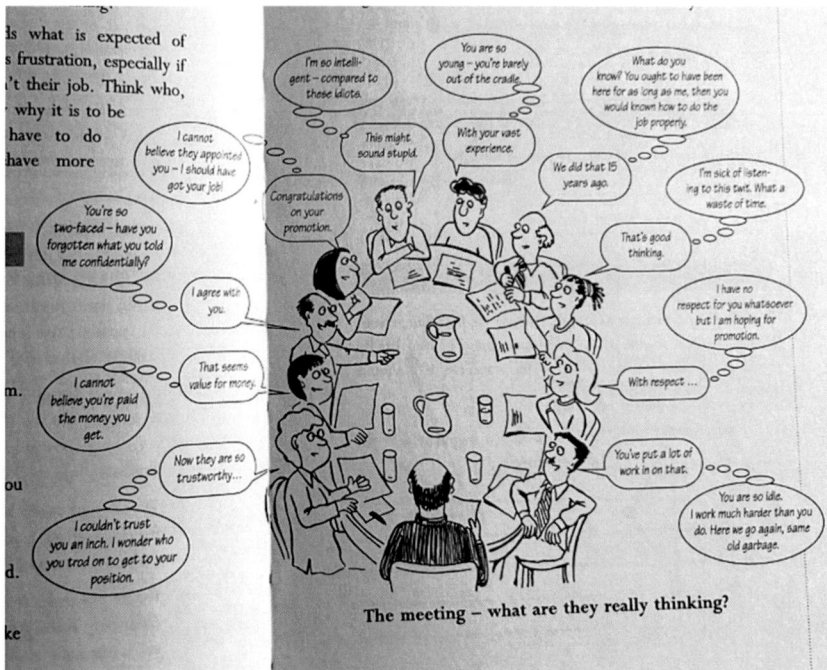

The meeting – what are they really thinking?

For example, someone might say:

- We trust you – (I would not trust you an inch I wonder who you have been chatting up to get your undeserved position.)
- That seems funny – (never heard anything so trite.)
- I agree with you – (you liar you are so two-faced. You forgot what you told me confidentially.)
- Congratulations on your new promotion – (It should have been me who got that job, more male chauvinism?)

34. Leadership

Stay away from negative people. They have a problem for every solution.

Do you know, or have you known, any negative people? At present we are in the midst of a political leadership contest, some are choosing a new leader. What sort of leader do you consider to be positive? Are they a good leader if they share your values?

What memories do you have of leaders in your life? Maybe a teacher at school, that you think was a good leader and helped you to understand, maybe they had a positive attitude when working with you and made you feel good about yourself and you looked forward to their lessons. You may have experienced other leaders when you were in the Scouts, Guides, Cubs, Brownies or other similar youth groups, remember them?

Think of the managerial leaders you have experienced when you were in either paid or voluntary work. Have you been on committees and seen individuals fighting for power? How would you describe them? There are four main types of leaders, psychologically:

The Visionary leader – the designer.

An architect of change, your sceptical approach questions everything. You have x-ray vision, intellectually ingenious, can see power bases, and power structures, have self-power awareness so you don't need to be competitive. Your own need for support – you need to praise people more often.

The Traditional leader –the stabiliser.

Decisive, follow-through commitment and have common sense. Keeps traditions, maintains a sense of permanence. Likes official rituals and present giving. Likes people to get to the point quickly, becomes irritated with wafflers. Your need for support may get hung up on laws, rules, need to work on your people skills

The Negotiating leader – the practical diplomat.

Adaptable, gets the jobs done. Enjoys and seeks change. Superb negotiator on such things as policies, procedures and personnel. Your need for support – is to have people around you to remind you of the other unpleasant jobs you need to do.

The Charismatic leader – the participated democrat.

Personal charisma, commitment, good at relating to people, good interpersonal skills, draw out active individuals, a natural empathiser and optimist. Your need for support – you are likely to put others before yourself, neglect your own health and you dislike formal authoritative people.

Thinking of the leaders you rated highly, which category would you now put him or her in?

The above types taken from *Leadership Skills for Success* published 1997 by Ward Lock – Jean Civil

Success is the ability to go from one failure to another, with no loss of enthusiasm.

35. Time Is Your Life

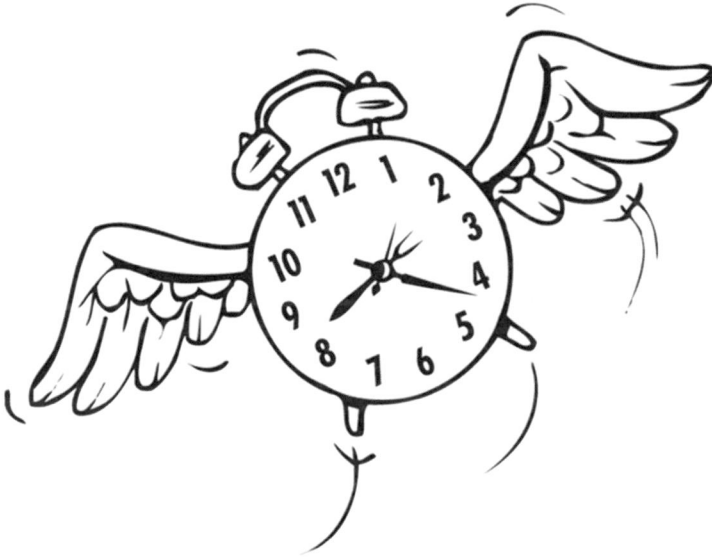

Life is made up of time. Waste your time and you waste your life.

There is a particular psychologist, Eric Berne, whose analytic theory is named Transactional Analysis. Many of you may have studied or have heard about it.

He stated how people spend their lives structuring their time in a certain way.

What do you do with your time? Are you able to sit and simply reflect? Do you feel some compulsion to fill every idle moment with some task or activity? Do you say frequently to others that you never have time to do things for yourself? You are so busy because you work, got children, feel stressed, not slept, got an idle partner! In TA, time structuring is divided into six categories:

Withdrawal

This may be mental, like when your mind wanders to more interesting things or physical, you stay on the outside of a gathering.

Rituals

Are like behaviour programmes; "Hello", "Good Morning", where you are 'doing the right thing'; you are 'in step' with everybody else. How are you? Fine! (when you are not).

Pastimes

Ways of getting to know, people without commitment to friendship or any real intimacy; like small talk in the village hall, parties, talking about the weather, clothes, the price of beer, Trump and so on.

Games

These are really interesting, games people play. More of this next time.

They appear OK and are plausible at a social level but all kinds of feelings and thoughts may be lurking just underneath the surface, like ulterior transactions. Games are played because they have a 'pay off' – the real purpose for the game.

Activities

Are ways of structuring time to get to know people a little more and getting something done. Like serving on a committee, going to church, bar duty, gardening, cooking dinner, washing up, being in the pantomime. Within activities, withdrawal, rituals and pastimes may be found, as are many games.

Intimacy

Involves genuine caring and is free of games and exploitation. It is clean, genuine – has no phoniness about it and is at a deeper level than all the other kinds of time structuring. It is how we describe real contact between people. It may be fleeting or last for years. In intimate relationships people are vulnerable and may feel frightened by the contact. It may feel safer for them to engage in other time-structuring ploys and many people use them to avoid intimacy. Do you?

36. The Psychology of Parenting

"I was treated so badly as a child that there is no way I would put my child through that, so yes I suppose I do spoil her. I was never praised, I was never touched or hugged, I just want the best for her."

Do you recognise similar thoughts and feelings, or have you said this to yourself?

Are you a parent? If you are – what sort of parent are you?

Parenting styles can affect everything from how much your child weighs to how they feel about themselves. It is important to ensure that parenting styles support healthy growth and development because the way we interact with our children influences them for the rest of their life. Researchers have identified four types of parenting styles: Each style takes a different approach to raising children. They are –

1. Authoritarian
2. Authoritative
3. Permissive
4. Uninvolved

1. **Authoritarian Parents** – think that kids should be seen and not heard; that only their way is the right way; they are unlikely to take the child's feelings into consideration. May respond with "because I say so" when the child asks why. They use punishment to make the kid feel sorry. Children of authoritarian parents are likely to grow up following the rules, but at a price, and also making good liars in their effort to avoid punishment. May grow up to feel anger towards their parents, have low self-esteem, because their feelings and thoughts are not valued.

2. **Authoritative Parents** – work at maintaining a positive relationship with their child. They explain the reasons behind their rules but take their child's

feelings into consideration. If you think that this is your style, you invest time and energy into preventing behaviour problems before they start. You have clear boundaries. You also use positive discipline strategies to reinforce good behaviour, like praise and reward. Children of authoritative parents tend to be happy and successful. They're also more likely to be good at making decisions and evaluating safety risks on their own. Researchers have found kids who have authoritative parents are most likely to become happy responsible adults who feel comfortable in expressing their opinions.

3. **Permissive Parents** – set rules but rarely enforce them. Don't follow through, or give clear consequences and think that the child will learn best if they don't interfere. They're quite forgiving and they adopt an attitude of "kids will be kids." When they do use consequences, they may not make those consequences stick. They might give privileges back if the child begs or cries or they may allow a child to get out of 'time-out' early if they promise to be good. Permissive parents usually want to take on more of a friend role than a parent role. They often encourage their children to talk with them about their problems, but they usually don't put much effort into discouraging poor choices or bad behaviour. Kids who grow up with permissive parents are more likely to struggle academically. They may exhibit more behavioural problems as they don't appreciate authority and rules. They often have low self-esteem and may report a lot of sadness. They're also at a higher risk for health problems, like obesity, some permissive parents struggle to organise their time and establish a routine so don't limit junk food intake.

4. **Uninvolved Parents** – don't ask their child about school or homework, rarely know where their child is, or with whom, and probably don't spend much time with them, choosing to go for fun, adult pursuits rather than following their child's interests. They do get involved occasionally to shine themselves, but become unreliable when it comes to prioritising their child's time. Many parents have a career desire and a preferred lifestyle which may mean farming out the children to paid carers, nannies, lots of clubs, private activities and hobbies or residential public schools. Uninvolved parents tend to make few rules expecting children to raise themselves. They don't devote much time or energy into meeting children's basic needs. They may be neglectful but it's not always intentional. A parent with mental health issues or substance abuse problems, for

example, may not be able to care for a child's physical or emotional needs on a consistent basis. At other times, uninvolved parents may lack knowledge about child development. Sometimes, they are simply overwhelmed with other problems, like work, paying bills, or managing a home. Children with uninvolved parents are likely to struggle with self-esteem issues and tend to perform poorly in school. They also exhibit frequent behaviour problems and rank low in happiness.

The studies are clear, however, that authoritative parenting is the best parenting style. With dedication and commitment to being the best parent you can be, you can maintain a positive relationship with your child while still establishing your authority in a healthy manner. Your child will reap the benefits of your authoritative style. Sometimes parents don't fit into just one category, so don't despair if there are times or areas where you tend to be permissive and other times when you're more authoritative. I still feel guilty, sometimes also regretful, for having been a serious professional woman and having a nanny!

Working with the parents in Midsummer's Night Green has been such a pleasure watching and admiring some of their parenting skills. As well as their supportive and caring skills towards me. Thank you, all parents, (and children) for making this event such fun.

37. Sexuality at Work

After six years of researching into Sexuality at work and finding that 90% of managers are affected by their sexuality at work, I am surprised that people are surprised.

Want to know more, then try the following questionnaires which were based on my research findings? These are taken from my book *Sexuality at Work; how does it affect you?* published 1998 by Batsford Business Books.

In fact, during my research I wondered if anyone went to work to work!

Questionnaire 1: What kind of role model are you as a manager?
Answer in Yes or No.

1. Does any of your staff think that you are sexually involved with someone?

   _____

2. Does your behaviour suggest that you have a favourite?

   _____

3. Do you spend more time with some staff than others because you are sexually attracted to them?

   _____

4. Have you been promoted because of some sexual liaison with a person of influence?

   _____

5. Have any of your staff commented to you about other people's sexual relationships or behaviour, expecting you to address the difficulty but you have ignored their request?

_____

6. Have you witnessed sexual behaviour that seems inappropriate for the workplace but have refrained from commenting on it?

_____

7. Are you aware of any member of staff having difficulty in working with their line manager because he or she (the line manager) is sexually involved with another colleague but ignored dealing with it?

_____

8. Are you experiencing your lines of communication being blocked because of someone's sexual involvement with another colleague but not addressed the situation?

_____

9. Have you avoided speaking to individuals directly about how their sexuality is affecting other colleagues?

_____

10. Does your staff mistrust you to be able to handle and address situations of a sexual nature?

_____

How did you score? More than 3 'Yes' answers and you are a poor role model of a manager. Your staff are likely to be affected negatively by your management style.

Now let us consider your sexuality.

As a manager have you ever found yourself experiencing any of the following situations? See Questionnaire 2.

Have you been aware of the sexuality of others and wished that you were able to manage those situations more effectively? See Questionnaire 3.

Questionnaire 2: Your sexuality

Have you ever: Yes   No

1. Preferred to be at work rather than at home because you are sexually involved with someone? (Sexually involved would be sexually intimate or hoping to be.)

2. Promoted people to whom you are sexually attracted?

3. Promoted anyone with whom you have had or are having a sexual relationship?

4. Demoted anyone to whom you are sexually attracted?

5. Demoted anyone with whom you have had or are having a sexual relationship?

6. Had an affair with a colleague or client? (An affair would be termed as a sexual relationship you may or may not wish other colleagues or partners to know about.)

7. Found that if you had an affair it negatively affected the way in which you worked?

8. Had time off work because of the effect of a sexual relationship?

9. Appointed someone to whom you are sexually attracted?

10. Deliberately not appointed someone to whom you were attracted for whatever reason?

How did you score?

More than three 'Yes' answers? Your sexuality is likely to be influencing you at work and your staff may be adversely affected by your behaviour.

My research offers two possible reasons for the situations outlined above:

Either managers are worried about the possibility of starting a relationship, especially when a present partnership is in any kind of difficulty, or they are anxious about being able to work with someone who sexually arouses them.

Now think about the people with whom you work.

Questionnaire 3: Sexuality of others

Would you be able to;   Yes   No

1. Manage staff involved in a sexual relationship if you received a complaint?
2. Challenge someone about sexual innuendoes?
3. Address complaints of sexual harassment?
4. Handle the conflict between staff if a sexual relationship was involved?

5. Deal with an emotional male or female who wishes to discuss their personal concerns about an affair which has ended?
6. Work comfortably with someone of a different sexual orientation from yourself?
7. Set up support systems for people who are HIV positive?

8. Initiate and complete a policy for dealing with sexual relationships at work?
9. Support a pregnant, unmarried, member of staff who claims that another, married member of your staff is the father of the unborn child?

10. Discuss with your senior manager his or her sexual behaviour, which you think, is affecting the workings of the organisation?

Enjoy your sexuality. It is a vital element of your being.

FINAL CHECKLIST

S	Sexual feelings happen at work
E	Early sexual messages can affect people's sexual attitudes
X	Explain that harassment will not be tolerated
U	Understand that staff have difficulties with sexuality between colleagues
A	Address complaints from staff about others' behaviour
L	Love is fine; lust is not
I	Implement a sexual harassment policy
T	Talk to staff when you believe their relationship is negatively affecting others
Y	You need to realise that some women staff may feel marginalised
A	Always be confidential about harassment disclosures
T	Try to relax when discussing items of a sexual nature. Listen with empathy to staff's concerns about sexual behaviour at work
W	Watch your language to prevent offence
O	Organise a policy that covers relationships at work
R	Remember that male and female chauvinism still exists
K	Keep a record of complaints about sexual issues

Sexuality at Work [(ISBN 0 7134 8370 9) – by Batsford Business Books] 1999 Author Jean Civil

Celebrating

38. Cultural Rituals

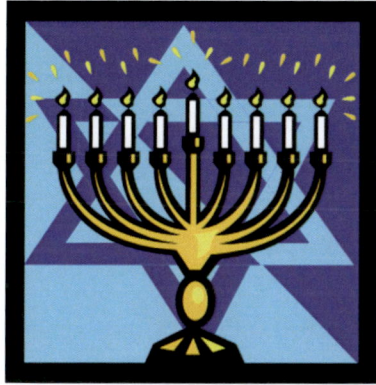

What celebrations do you have in your life? Whatever religious or non-religious beliefs do you now hold and follow? Almost everyone, as a child will have had some messages and scripts about their family and their cultural rituals. As you grew up did you feel misled, even lied to, did you ever lose trust in the significant people who were then in your life?

You may have heard stories; even lies, about certain family members. The then word 'illegitimate', often cropped up in such revelations. It is a word hardly ever used now, describing someone, usually used then with tones of judgement, shame and a closely guarded, kept secret, not so many years ago. Reflecting back to your childhood stories, of whatever kind, did you in later years feel, angry, hurt, let down, that an adult that you trusted did actually lie to you?

Let us look at the ritual of Father Christmas or Santa Clause, visiting many children to give them presents.

How old were you when you first wondered about Santa?

Substitute the word Santa with the name of your particular 'religious' or special person, that you might have been told about in your childhood. Santa was St Nicolas.

Were the stories that you heard at school true, was the story of Santa true or was it all a fib, was it really parents or steppos that bought you the presents? Did 'a grown up' parent, or some significant adult in your young life explain or answer your questions?

I remember asking an uncle who brought me up, whom I really liked and trusted "Father Christmas cannot be true can he, because there are so many children in the world for him to give them all presents on Christmas Eve, he wouldn't be able to do all of that in one night."

I received a very understandable answer that of course I was right he could not possibly do that all on his own; he had loads of other little Father Christmases to help him, which also delivered. Right, sorted. I believed him because I trusted him.

According to several academics, parents, and general Santa critics, there are about eight long years of lies that could have damaged the development and relationship that children have with their parents.

Santa Claus remains a controversial figure among many scientists and parents. There are countless books on the subject, including *The Myths that Stole Christmas*, which claims that the Santa legend is bad for kids. The main argument is, unsurprisingly, that telling kids about a magical figure who delivers presents to children around the world on Christmas Eve is a *lie*. This lie may be backed by good intentions, but it is a lie nonetheless, one that will inevitably unravel at some point during a child's development. Figuring out the truth can be traumatic for a child, this argument goes, and will project the message that children can't trust what their parents tell them. Furthermore, lying in order to encourage good behaviour is *manipulative* and encourages children to behave well for the wrong reasons.

There is some evidence that rewards (like Christmas gifts) undermine children's motivation. So maybe relying on Santa or an elf to promote good behaviour isn't the best strategy if you want your kids to be well behaved all year round. But there is no evidence suggesting that learning the truth about Santa is traumatic for a lot of children—or that it leads to trust issues between kids and their parents.

It might be good advice for parents to stop being so dishonest with their kids about other issues. In a recent study on parental lying, the researchers asked adults if they had been lied to by their parents when growing up. Those people who were lied to the most by their parents were more likely to lie back to their parents. More importantly, they also had higher levels of psychosocial maladjustment.

Dr Drew Curtis's study on lying about Santa, asked college students how often their parents had promoted the myth of Santa Clause, and asked them how they felt about it and how was their relationship with their parents. Curtis found that most reported that their parents had lied about Santa a lot. They also said that they viewed their parents' Santa lies as being somewhat dishonest. Fortunately for parents, he found that there was no link between how many Santa lies had been told and how good a relationship people had with their parents now.

You can be a good role model, or you can be a bad role model. Your choice. However, being a dishonest parent about other issues may be setting the stage for your kids to have a tough time ahead. 'Monkey does what monkey sees, or hears, or feels.' Childhood scripts may still deeply affect many of us. Do you still feel hurt about a lie or something that was said to you when you were a child? Try asking the same question to your family and friends.

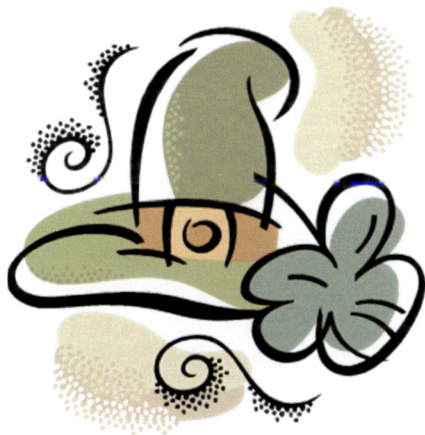

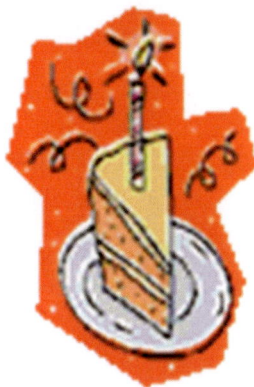

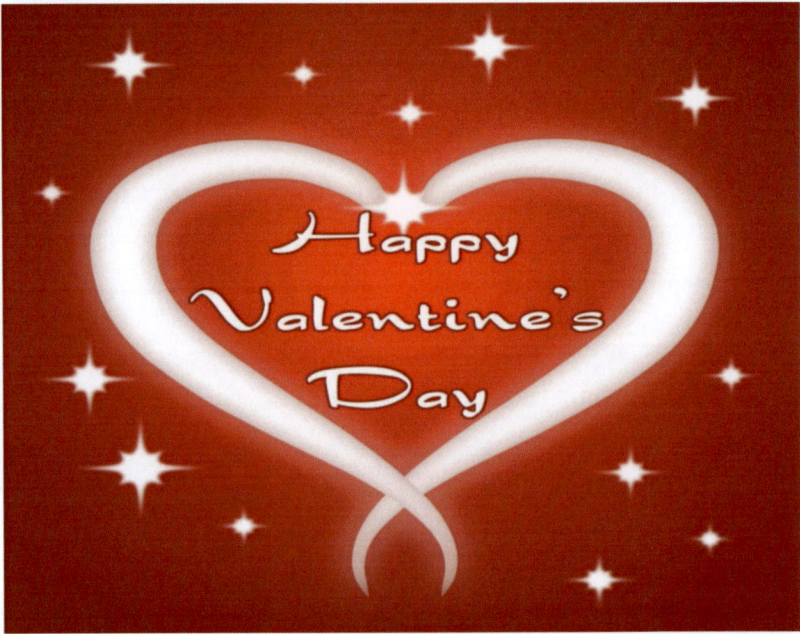

39 B St Valentine's Day and Love

So, we are now in February with Valentine's Day to look forward to, well for some of us that is, as evidence shows that many people who are single and unattached on Valentine's Day may become depressed by being caught up with the hype of love and advertising of the day.

After the third Monday in January, that has now gone, which is the saddest day of the year, (that is why it is called blue Monday,) as it is the most depressing and most likely day for suicide attempts; Sadly, Valentine's Day is also a significant date for similar mind thinking behaviour.

However, for the majority of people, the day is joyous and a time for romance and an opportunity to give gifts to lovers, husbands, wives, partners, relations or to share time affectionately with genuine friends.

Valentine's Day was initiated on the day that St Valentine, who was a Priest or a Bishop died in the third century, on 14 Feb 269 A.D. (or CD) having been born in 226, so he was around 42 years of age.

In terms of linking him with love, there are many legends, one of which is that St Valentine when he was a priest, he encouraged and married Christian couples and defied the Roman Emperor by secretly performing marriage ceremonies. This meant that many young men had an excuse for not enrolling or joining the army as married men were considered not to be good soldiers as they would be thinking about their wives and families when they were married.

I love you. Love is most likely to be expressed as a positive emotion with vastly differing degrees of intensity. We can say we love the sun, the sea, a particular food or a particular piece of music or a person. Many men and women pledge love to a spouse or partner or until death do us part.

So, what is love and can I love in different ways?

There are four Greek words: *Eros*, *Storge*, *Philia*, and *Agape*. All meaning love, in order of writing, Romantic love, Family love, Brotherly love, and Divine love.

Eros (Pronounced: AIR-ohs) is the Greek word for sensual or romantic love. The term originated from the mythological Greek goddess of love, sexual desire, physical attraction, and physical love.

Storge (Pronounced: STOR-jay) This Greek word describes family love, the affectionate bond that develops naturally between parents and children, and brothers and sisters.

Philia (Pronounced: FILL-ee-uh) is the type of intimate love the powerful emotional bond seen in deep friendships. Philia is the most general type of love, encompassing love for fellow humans, care, respect, and compassion for people in need. The concept of brotherly love that unites most of us, but not necessarily as we know.

Agape (Pronounced: Uh-GAH-pay) Agape love is perfect, unconditional, sacrificial, and pure.

While Romantic love has three elements:

1. **Attachment:**

This is the need to be cared for and be with the other person. Physical contact and approval are also important components of attachment.

2. **Caring:**

We are likely to show that we care by valuing the other person's happiness and needs as much as our own.

3. **Intimacy:**

This means both mentally and physically we experience romantic love by sharing private thoughts, feelings, and physical desires with the other person.

4. **Self-love:**

This is also very important in the process of good mental health and psychotherapy.

No, it is not selfish to love yourself. It is about forgiving ourselves, warts and all.

"Love thy neighbour as thyself." No wonder that so many of us are so awful and rotten to our neighbours, as few of us love ourselves! Do you love yourself?

Well, who do you love, who loves you, who do you love that doesn't love you, who loves you but you don't love them? Can you love more than one person?

Do you have different kinds of love?

How do you behave when you feel someone does not love you?

What a lot of questions. What about answers, are there any?

Yes, one answer is to start by loving yourself. Then you can love others.

When you let go of who you are, you are able to find who you can be. A Buddhist saying. Hence, Valentine's Day presents us with the many opportunities we have to express our love outwardly with cards, (maybe some secretly) flowers and/or chocolates, maybe going out for a romantic dinner in a couple or with a group of loving genuine friends.

39. Giving and Receiving Presents

Do you find that you prefer to give presents rather than to receive them?

Your mental state is important in both of these transactions. The way in which you accept a present can bring joy or misery to the giver or you may show your embarrassment apologizing at your lack of reciprocation or thoughtfulness.

Therefore, whatever is the occasion, family, friends, working occasions, any religious celebration, we need to be aware of how our mental state can affect others and ourselves.

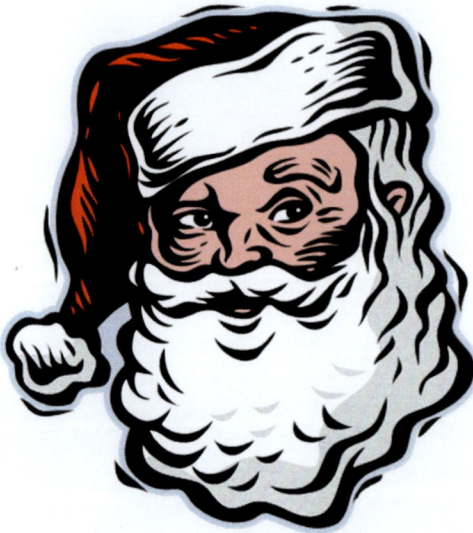

Christmas, for many people is the time of year of maybe giving and receiving gifts. So what did you say to yourself or think when asked which do you prefer giving rather than receiving? Some do! When receiving a gift, do you feel embarrassed that you have not had the same thoughtfulness that a friend may have shown towards you?

Pre-Christmas is that time of year when some people start getting excited by the prospects of hunting through the shops on the high street, or through endless internet sites, searching for all those perfect gifts for loved ones. Well, some get excited, whilst others hate it, are full of anxiety dreading the prospect every Christmas time, believing that Christmas is about celebrating Christ's birth rather than commercial hype. So that begs the question, why do we do it?

To understand this ritual, it's important to understand more about us as a species. Humans are a very social species, our success in living and working with each other has been shaped over millions of years of evolution. As a result, humans benefit far more by cooperating with one another rather than by only caring about themselves. Something that Charles Darwin struggled to explain, as his theory of natural selection suggests that we should only be interested in our own survival, which is why many people believe and act on sayings like 'survival of the fittest', or the richest!

'Giving' has long been a favourite subject for studies on human behaviour, with psychologists, anthropologists, economists and marketers. Many psychologists have found that giving gifts is a surprisingly complex and important part of human interaction, helping to define relationships and strengthen bonds with family and friends. Indeed, psychologists say it is often the giver, rather than the recipient, who reaps the biggest psychological gains from a gift.

When you give a gift, it makes you feel generous, it may make you feel in control, it's good for your self-esteem and it's good for the relationship, because maybe you come to know the person even better. Gifts do not have to be expensive, they can be inviting someone for a meal, babysitting, offering a car lift or sending a caring card.

40. Saying Thank You

'You shouldn't have bought me a present! You didn't need to have done that!' Have you ever said something similar to someone giving you a gift? Have you ever given someone a present that you have taken a lot of trouble about, choosing it, or making it and taking time and trouble to wrap it attractively? Only to have the receiver discount you by saying something like 'Oh, I didn't get you anything' or 'I didn't think we were doing presents.'

So, the next time you are given a gift, try not to discount the giver, just say thank you, like you do when you are given a compliment (as if)! As we say "It's the thought that counts!"

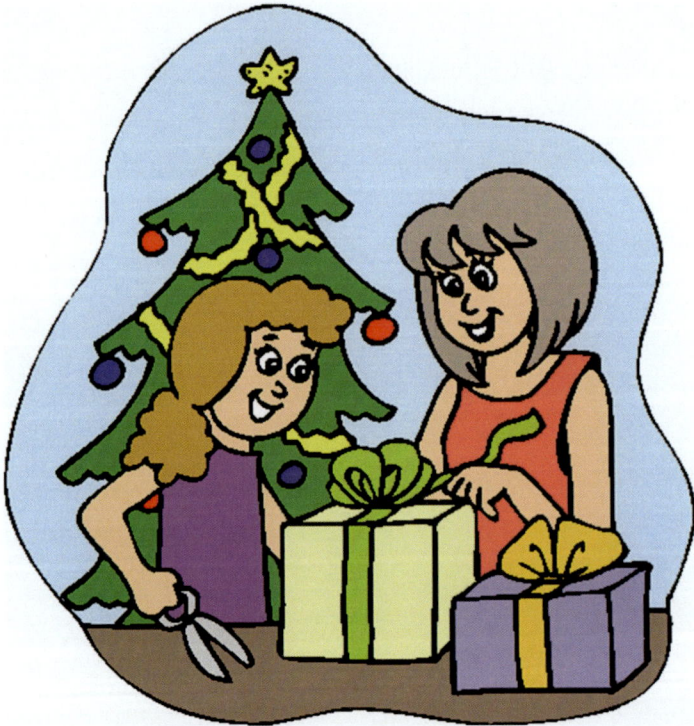

Hence, no more faux pars like

Oh, I already have one

It is the wrong size

I hate purple flowers

Yellow has never suited me but thanks anyway.

Smile, make eye contact and say thank you, or lie and say how much you like it, even though you may be thinking differently.

That way you will both feel mentally at peace with yourselves.

41. Making New Year Resolutions

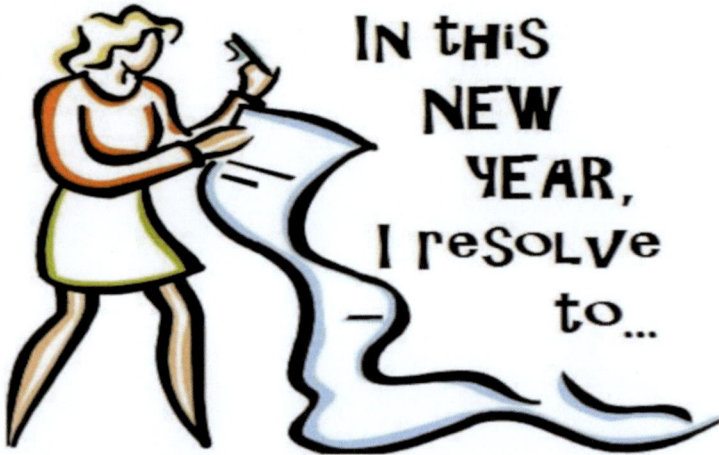

Yes, I always make one, even though I know that research has shown that about half of all adults make **New Year's resolutions**. However, fewer than 10% manage to keep them for more than a few months.

Why on earth do 50% of people make them? Many psychologists are most likely to say that is the allure of starting again from scratch. The beginning of the year offers a fresh start and a clean slate.

The idea of our bettering ourselves is another motivator. Most of us have a natural bent towards self-improvement; so many resolutions are about a healthier body or more likely these days, a healthy mind with more emphasis being placed on trying to get help when you are mentally distressed. More celebrities are now talking about their depression, secret fears and behaviours.

As well as it being about tradition, the ritual of setting New Year's resolutions is believed to go back as far as Babylonian times. It's said that Julius Caesar started the tradition of making resolutions on January 1st as a way to honour the Roman mythical god Janus, whose two faces allowed him to look back into the past year and forward to the new year. Romans mostly made morality-based resolutions, such as seeking forgiveness from their enemies.

To change our behaviour, we have to change our attitude. For some people a radical illness can change our behaviour overnight. The death of a loved one from an illness, heart attack, cancer, or your own medical diagnosis, can be radical in our changing our ways. A pregnancy can mean giving up alcohol or smoking when previously it was a struggle to stop.

Be realistic. You need to begin by making resolutions that you can keep. If you want to reduce your alcohol intake, do it every other day, don't immediately go teetotal. The same principle can be applied to exercise or eating more healthily.

Do one at a time. One of the easiest routes to failure is to have too many resolutions.

Be SMART – That is, they need to be; Specific, Measurable, Achievable, Realistic and Timed. Maybe tell someone about your resolution.

You may like to join up with someone who shares your resolution.

Maybe wanting to make resolutions is a good thing it gives us hope and a certain level of belief in our ability to change and be more of who we really want to be.

Here is a magic wand, what would you like to be?

Now go and be it.

My Mind Makes Me Mentally Well

Does yours?

42. Psychological Games People Play

This is not about the importance of sport and exercise for our good mental health but about the psychological games that many people and we play.

Be aware of them, realise how you get hooked, finding yourself dependant on partners that control, bully, abuse you, and mentally destroy your self-belief, confidence, self-respect and love. Friends, family, neighbours, school and work colleagues can also abuse you. Of course, it is not just partners.

So, neither is it about table games like bridge. On one occasion, I was told that an article that I had written about 'the games people play', which she had read, had upset an elderly woman, who has since died, as the person thought I meant bridge, of which she was an expert. Intimacy and manipulation is often the reason for our playing games, and we play games in order to avoid intimacy. She was hurt and thought that I meant she was manipulative.

Hence, that is the reason that I am taking the trouble of explaining how.

Perhaps the person telling me the story of how distressed the elderly woman was may have been playing the game of 'got you' with me.

So yes, we play psychological games in order to avoid intimacy and to get into our bad feelings. Games are time-consuming. They usually cause trouble. They are relationship wreckers and misery producers.

The word 'game' does not necessarily imply fun or even enjoyment. It certainly does not mean bridge or similar board games which are so helpful and important to so many individuals who would be lost without the wonderful friendship they have with other players.

Often the names of the games sound funny, but the negative affect that psychological games can cause, are not. They make us mentally ill.

Games like:

"Why don't you" – **"yes but!"** – offering ideas but the response is almost always "yes but". Who springs to mind that you know who does that? Teachers, social workers and medics know this game well when they try to help.

"Look at what you've made me do now!" – I am thinking of a child or adult dropping an ice cream on them self, then blames you. In fact, it is also another named game.

'The Blame game!' – Do you do that? Do you always find a reason why it is not your fault? Guess you probably have to have the last word as well.

"Poor me!" – Everything goes wrong in my life and now my cat has died. Do you know someone who plays this game with you or perhaps it's you? Do you play it, by always moaning about how hard life has been for you and how you have suffered?

"I'm more important than you" – those whose minds think like that are so sad. They are controlling and often a narcissist, not a team player, disliked for their behaviour, they are usual bossy, even bullying, stubborn, do not want change to their area of importance and want only their own way. Who is coming to your mind in your life?

'Blemish!' Does not matter what you do for someone you think and feel that the person in your mind is always looking for your mistake or finding fault with whatever idea or attitude you express. They will always point out something that is, or could go, wrong.

"Kick me!" – do you set up games and situations, so that you will feel rejected. We almost all of us have a 'racket feeling' or a negative place that we can slip into because of what happened to us in our earlier lives. Rejection is a common one. It is mine. Rackets are comfortable bad feelings. Comfortable because they are familiar you have been there before, bad because hurt.

Uproar – a sexual game, you or partner bring about to enjoy the initiates of a row to making up.

Wooden leg! If it wasn't for my wooden leg, I could have done that! Using anything as a reason for procrastinating. Who do you know who does that?

"Ain't it awful 'ere?" – moan, moan, moan

NIGYYSOB! (Now I've Got You, You Son of a Bitch) this game is like

NIGTTLAY! (Now I'm going to throw the lot at you)

"I told you so" – so that they can feel superior and back in control

Many games are played which are self-explanatory in their titles, for instance,

"Let you and the other person fight".

You can make up your own titles for the psychological games played in your home and social life. One of my closest women friends had a game called 'Knickers'. When her partner asked her "Where is my (whatever) …" she would reply with "Where are my knickers?"

The golden rule is **don't collaborate with the game,** remember that once you hit the ball back, you are in the other person's game.

Address the games by saying:

"That sounds as if you are playing the 'blame game'."

Ask yourself who plays psychological games with you. Also, with whom do you play psychological games in order for you to get what you want or avoid intimacy?

Stop it, just ask for what you want, say what you are thinking or feeling or how you want to behave.

However good you are – people cannot read your mind.

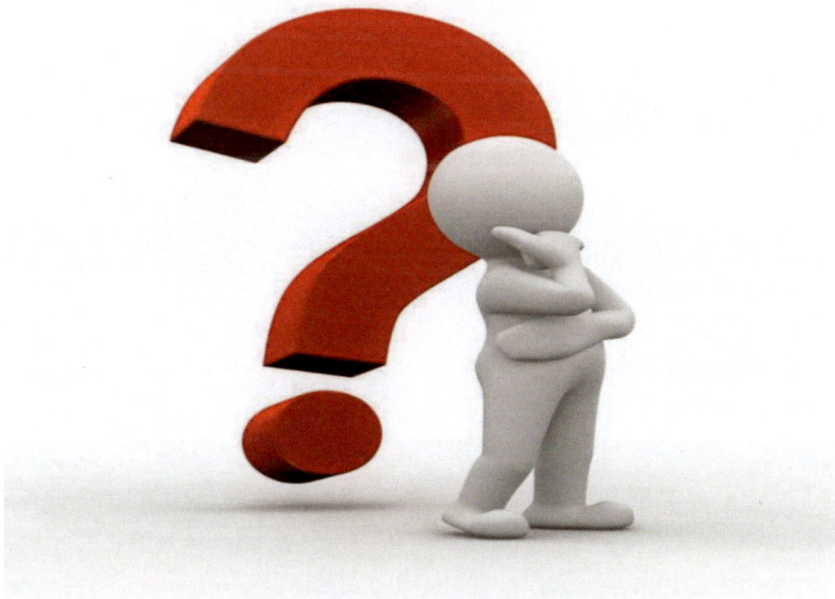

43. Volunteering

One of the main reasons for individuals volunteering is often to make money for charity but for some to meet people of their own age in an area. However, what is special about this chapter is that it can help us all to achieve many of the things that we are discussing, friendship, happiness, belonging, so avoiding loneliness and depression and achieving good mental health.

The benefits of volunteering are well known – making a difference, giving back to the community, and developing new skills for example but there is less clarity about what psychological aspects make a volunteer. However, it is thought that;

1. Retirement – there are a lot of retired people in many resorts and certain parts of the country attract them. Volunteers live longer and are healthier, they are happier and healthier than non-volunteers. In fact, later in life, volunteering is even more beneficial for one's health than exercising and eating well. Older people who volunteer remain physically functional longer, have more robust psychological well-being, and live longer. However, older people who volunteer are almost always people who volunteered earlier in life. Health and longevity gained from volunteering usually comes from establishing meaningful volunteer roles before you retire.

2. Loneliness – Volunteering establishes strong relationships. Despite all of the online connections that are available at our fingertips, people are lonelier now than ever before. A study in 2010 reported that prevalence of loneliness is at an all-time high, with about one in three adults aged 45 or older categorised as lonely. Online connections, with old relationships help but are not very helpful in establishing lasting, new ones. Working alongside people who feel as strongly as you do about supporting a particular cause creates strong relationships with others. It isn't just beneficial for making new friendships, either: if you volunteer alongside members of your family this strengthens family bonds based in 'doing' your values. Children who volunteer with their parents are more likely to become adults who volunteer.

3. Career – Volunteering can be good for your career. People who volunteer make more money, partially because the relationships people create while volunteering can lead to a financial benefit. In 1973, Johns Hopkins and sociologist Mark Granovetter described the important role of 'weak ties'. Weak ties are those relationships that are outside of one's close-knit social network. These relationships may bring new opportunities. Volunteering has long been viewed as a way to create new 'weak tie' connections that may lead to career opportunities.

4. Young people – so many young people face fewer jobs in the current climate. The latest findings in a recent survey showed that 70% of the 2021 young people involved in the research were likely and willing to participate in social action in the future, but 41% said that they weren't sure how to get involved – a clear opportunity to improve our communications with this young group. The analysts also classified the respondents into three groups based on their current, previous and intended participation in social action – they were either committed, potential or reluctant. Which are you?

5. Volunteering is good for society. It is certainly good for our village, as we have so many volunteers. These volunteers are committed to doing so many good things for us and participate in helping to meet the needs of people from all walks of life.

Here is a volunteer who opened his amazing precious Model railway up for the charity sale, asking for donations. Graham Ward, some will know him as the ogre in our last pantomime.

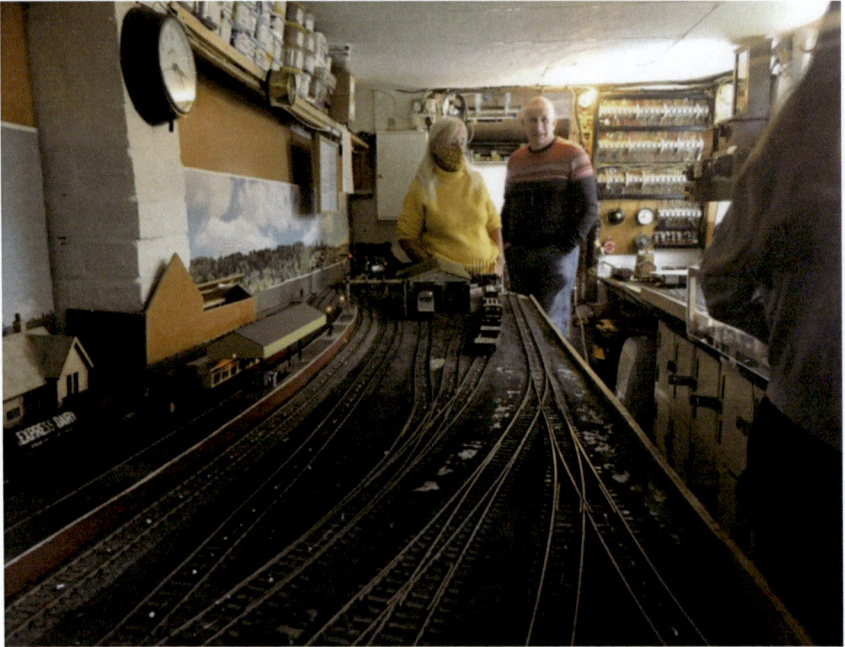

Volunteering for the Community Pantomime

"Three years to ninety years" – that is the answer, what is the question?

The question is "What is the age range of our cast in our voluntary Pantos?" What a motley crew they are from all walks of life.

Now here is another answer –

"International ice skater; Electrical engineer; Teacher trainer; University lecturer; Manager of building firm; Director of international sound company; Architect; Gynaecologist; Accountant; PE teacher; Nursery Nurse, Drama student; Plumber; Psychotherapist; Railway engineer; Nurse; Artist; Drama teacher; Photographer; Solicitor; Director of school travel; Sex therapist; Author; Brighton Bell driver, Pharmaceutical salesperson, Two Brighton Mayors and Vicar and a Rector." That is the answer and the question is – "What sort of jobs have the drama cast had or still have?"

Modern pantomime includes songs, gags, slapstick comedy and dancing. Pantos have gender-crossing actors and combine topical local humour with a story based on a well-known fairy tale. The most important part of all pantos is that in the story there are goodies and baddies but always the moral and the mantra at the end is that no matter what happens in the story *good always overcomes evil*. Pity it is not always true in real life.

Panto is a participatory form of theatre, in which the audience joins in. 'Oh yes they do.' Hence the instruction now is we want audience participation. The audience is expected to sing along with certain parts of the music and shout out well known panto phrases to the performers. Well known ones like "Oh yes, it is"; "Oh no it's not"; "It's behind you". Ogres and baddies usually think that they are so handsome so we expect the audience to shout out … "Oh no you're not". Most baddies in our lives are narcistic. Do you have anyone in mind?

Do you find that? So, when you see a pantomime be prepared to see lots of strange little people being all sorts of imaginary things. Most of all it also gives the children a chance to gain confidence, find and make long-lasting friendships and have the warm fuzzy feeling of being applauded.

Many 'old' faces will be recognised alongside lots of lovely fresh-faced children, both as leads and supporting actors are in our mindful feeling behaving fun panto and it gives many people lots of laughs. They do make me laugh working with such fun people. Almost all children are just so beautifully honest.

44. Ecology

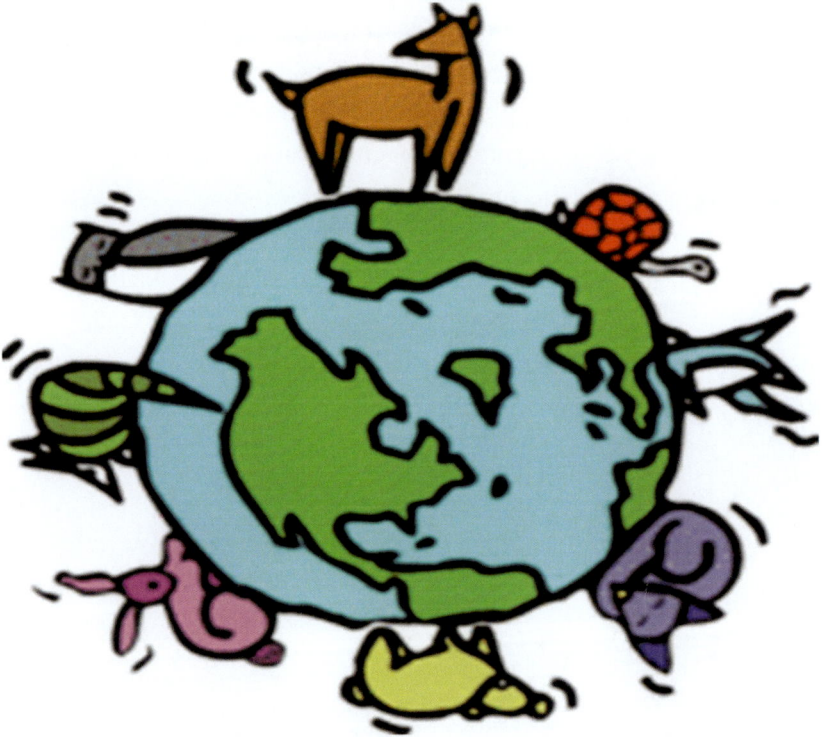

Ecology is a type of science that relates to the environment.

The suffix '-ology' simply means 'the study of'. Therefore, the term psychology means the study of the mind (the psyche) whilst 'ecology' means the study of the environment.

This may include organisms, animals and plant types. We need to be aware of how our individual actions affect the environment. The unnecessary overuse of polythene; dropping litter; caring for Beacon Hill Nature reserve and taking away all our rubbish when spending time on our beach and recycling.

Most of us though are ignorant about the complicated processes of global production and consumption. We have had precisely this contextual awareness stripped away from us. This ignorance isn't anyone's fault but it does mean, again, that most of us have developed some deeply grooved mental habits regarding how we behave impulsively interacting with the world of objects, that is to say how we use 'stuff'. We are interdependent.

Equally most of us are interdependent on each other. We also need to be aware of how our individual actions affect the minds of the people in our village community. Saying good morning, smiling, looking for the positive, instead of the negative in people, commending rather than criticising. Bothering to ask someone how they are and then really listening to their answer. Recognising how people will often contribute, if approached, to the so many ventures, projects and activities in our village, if asked. Not taking for granted the immense amount of work that so many individuals do voluntarily for other people.

45. Kindness

However clever you are, without kindness, you will never fulfil your full potential.

Kindness is contagious. When we're kind we inspire others to be kind and studies show that it actually creates a ripple effect that spreads outwards to our friends. Dopamine is the reward chemical that is released by the brain and makes us feel good as a result of something that we perceive as positive. Oxytocin, responsible for emotional warmth, reduces blood pressure and promotes other cardiovascular benefits. It also reduces levels of free radicals and inflammation, thus slowing ageing.

Be kind to yourself. This isn't always as easy as it sounds. Most of us are incredibly hard on ourselves. We need to pay attention about the thoughts we have about ourselves. We may think that we are boring, disliked, an outsider of a group, lacking in friends. If someone said to you, that you look fat, ugly, you're not liked, weird. If you had a friend who spoke to you like that, you would be wise to start keeping your distance.

Be kind to strangers. This will make you feel more connected to the world you live in and take your mind off your own troubles. Be kind to those you love. So many people are so busy that they can forget someone they love, even in their own family. A phrase I heard many years ago "Pub Angel, House Devil" rings true.

Becoming more environmentally aware, is a good way of being kind. Be kind online; choose your language carefully so that people are not hurt.

Be kind in your community. Stick up for people that you feel are being bullied or rejected. Give blood, if you are able; join the NHS organ donor register; write a letter to somebody with whom you have been out of touch. Be kind for free, the most generous acts of kindness may often involve your giving your time, listening, loving, rather than cash. Researcher Elizabeth Dunn found that those who spend money on others reported much greater happiness than those who spend it on themselves.

Giving to others reduces depression and improves well-being. Researchers found people can actually build up their compassion 'muscle' and respond to others' suffering with care and a desire to help.

Volunteering results in more health benefits than exercising or quitting smoking. Helping a neighbour, volunteering, or donating goods and services results in a helper's high. Volunteers live longer and tend to have fewer aches and pains.

"The smallest act of kindness is worth more than the grandest intention."

Oscar Wilde

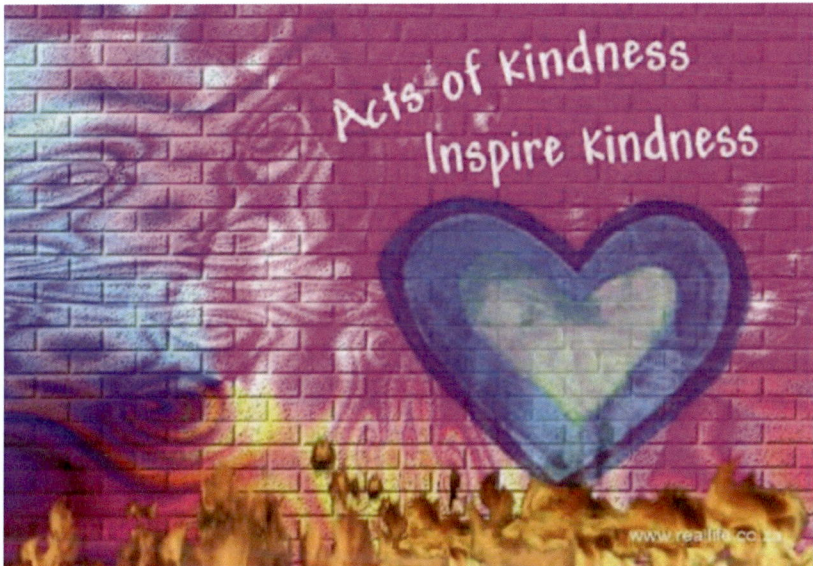

46. Happiness

What makes you happy? Before reading on, pause and think.

What makes one person happy could make someone else very miserable. We are all very different because many of us have such different values. Genuine friends often share values. Hence the reason and bedrock for their honest friendship. When we discuss happiness, we are referring to a person's enjoyment or satisfaction, which may last just a few moments or extend over the period of a lifetime. Happiness does not have to be expressed in order to be enjoyed – it is an internalised experience, varying in degrees, from mild satisfaction to wild euphoria.

There are numerous psychological theories on happiness. However, a main one is that there are three distinct kinds of happiness;

1. The pleasant life (a hedonistic search for pleasure)
2. The good life (engagement) and
3. The meaningful life

The first two are subjective but the third is more objective, hence – can happiness be measured? The United Nations seems to believe that it can, and released the *World Happiness Report*, which ranks countries by the self-reported happiness of its citizens. In 2016, the report listed Denmark as the happiest nation, followed by Switzerland and Iceland. The US was the 13th happiest country with the UK ranking 23rd. Nordic countries feature prominently as being amongst the happiest societies in the world.

A further finding is that we find more happiness if we belong and serve others. It is more worthwhile than in just seeking self-pleasures and desires. Another measurement at the University of Southern California, noticed a strange paradox involving money and happiness. Should a positive correlation exist between the two? We might expect citizens of developed countries to be happier than those of less prosperous nations. However, Richard Easterlin the award-winning economist discovered that this is not the case – rich people within countries tend to be happier than the poorest in the same country, but overall, those with little money are happier. He showed that when countries become wealthier the wealth contributes to social inequality and happiness levels do not rise across the population. As comedians say – money doesn't buy you happiness but it helps you to be miserable in comfort!

At a recent garden party. I asked people to answer quickly, "What makes you happy?"

It wasn't exactly qualitative analysis research, but it was interesting what common answers emerged. The sea, nature, good friends and family. My thoughts were the views of the sea and south downs from inside our house, my husband's humour and my son's smile.

"If you want others to be happy, practice compassion. If you want to be happy, practice compassion."

– Dalai Lama

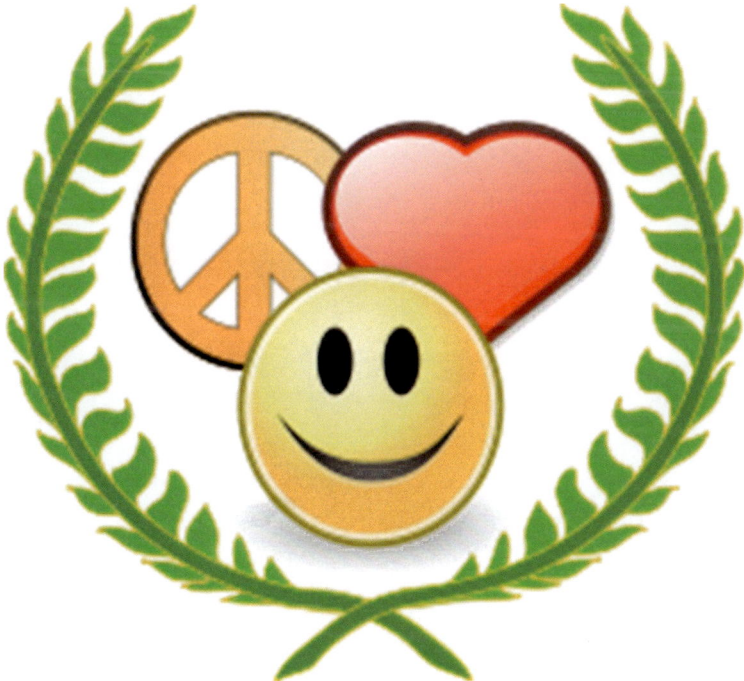

47. Dreams

We all dream. Some of us don't remember them.

Dreams are unopened letters from our subconscious.

Dreams can be associated with something that happened to us during that day.

They can be a way of warning you what is worrying you, behaviour that hurt you, something that was said that has left you feeling vulnerable, upset or angry.

Then there are reoccurring dreams. A trauma in your life that needs to be accepted.

A very close loving friend and an ex-student of mine who asked me if she could research dreams for her thesis for her Diploma in Counselling thesis, is Brenda Mallon, (author of The Dream Bible). She was on channel four TV and interviewed James Hewitt and many other celebrities on reoccurring dreams. James's dream was winning the Grand National, as he won, nobody cheered or clapped, all were silent. Analysis was that it would not matter what he achieved it was unlikely that he would regain peoples' approval.

Dreaming can also be a form of healing. Our dreams ask us to look at ourselves, the lives we lead, aspects that we may need to change and our relationships with others. They cover every part of our existence; physical, emotional, and spiritual. It is thought that they relay signals of impending illness that the subconscious translates into dreams. Every emotional feeling involves the release of neuropeptides which impacts on our physical wellbeing. Our dreams can reflect these emotional states and we can use them to become more aware of our inner lives.

Blocked emotions impact negatively on our immune system and make us more susceptible to illness. By expressing our feelings, we release these blockages which helps our immune system.

Sometimes we may dream of someone but that is not really the person that is worrying us. Even the subconscious cannot bring itself to show you.

How can we work with our dreams to aid physical, emotional and spiritual aspects of our lives? When you wake up, avoid rushing to the bathroom, lie still, keep your head in the same place and try to recall your dream. Remember dreams are symbolic. What do you think it is saying to you or warning you about?

48. On Laughter

Who makes you laugh?

Pause for a moment and think about it before reading on.

Who doesn't make you laugh?

What entertainment or hobbies make you laugh?

Initially for me I am thinking of those memorable laughing moments of being in the village hall, in the past, thinking of many fun people being on the stage; Mike in his grass skirt and coconut brassiere; John as Dame; Catherine in her orange socks as Magpie; the children dancing as Oompa-Loompas, some just being out of sync; watching Ted with his St Georges helmet on; hearing Peter's rendering of Albert and the Lion, or when he asked Susan for "line" in "When We Are Married"? Different things make different people laugh. Different strokes for different folks.

Which TV programmes make you laugh? Think of the comedy programmes, do you laugh at the Vicar of Dibley, Last of the Summer Wine, Dad's Army or are you more inclined to laugh at The Office or Friends or the Simpsons. Maybe your age has a bearing on your choice.

Here are some thoughts that you may or may not know about laughter.

Laughter isn't about jokes – Ask adults what makes them laugh, and most will tell you it's jokes and humour. But they would be wrong. Friends are more likely to make you laugh than jokes. Most people like quick repartee rather than long boring drawn out stories or jokes. Some people have the most wonderful laugh that is so contagious.

Pauline, Barbara, Debby, Richard, Sheila and many more.

Robert Provine, a psychologist found that we actually laugh most when talking to our friends. In fact, we're 30 times more likely to laugh at something when we are with other people. Intriguingly, within these conversations, we are still not laughing at jokes: we laugh at statements and comments that do not seem on the face of them to be remotely funny. It's a form of communication, not a reaction.

The psychology of laughter is telling us that laughter is less to do with jokes and is more to do with social behaviour which we use to show people that we like them and that we understand them.

Did you know that rats are ticklish?

Want to see a rat laugh? Then tickle it. Rats laugh, chimps laugh and so do dogs. But rats aren't laughing at jokes. They laugh when they're playing, in the same way humans do, to show that they're happy and to encourage bonding.

This is evidence that human laughter has evolved from playing, a behaviour seen in many other mammals.

The rats that played more, laughed more. And the ones that laughed more preferred to be around other rats that laughed. I prefer to be around people who laugh, do you?

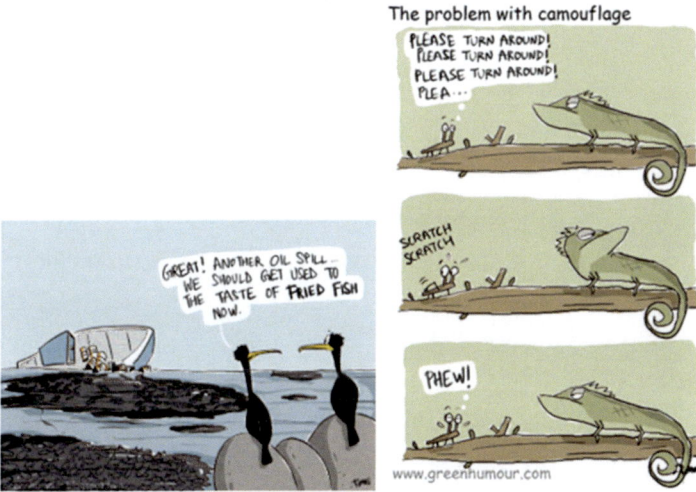

www.greenhumour.com

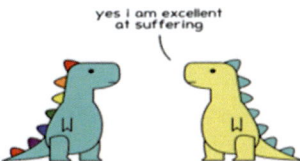

Your brain can tell the difference between deliberate and helpless laughter.

Do you know people who seem to force themselves to laugh with you or at you? Their laughter feels false and phoney or you just feel that they are being sycophantic or perhaps polite? Not only does your brain automatically tell the difference, but listening to staged laughter produces greater activity in an area called the anterior medial prefrontal cortex. It's known to be involved in understanding other people's emotions.

It shows that we automatically try to comprehend someone's deliberate laughs, even when not instructed to do so.

Laughter is catching.

Our brain scans also reveal that laughter is contagious, you can see the brain responding to the laughter by preparing the facial muscles to join in.

The more that someone shows a contagious response to laughter, the better they are at telling whether a laugh is real or forced.

This seems to suggest that joining in when you hear laughter is more than just contagion – it may be helping you to understand what that laughter means.

People you know are funnier.

People find jokes funnier if they think they were told by a famous comedian.

"Two snowmen are standing in a field. One says to the other: 'Funny, I can smell carrots too.'." – Even on paper it's funnier when you think it's coming from Eric Morecombe (or your favourite comedian) rather than Jamie Oliver.

Relationships last longer when you laugh.

Prof Bob Levenson a psychologist, asked couples to discuss something about their partner that annoyed them – a touchy subject indeed.

However, the couples that used laughter and smiling not only felt better immediately but they also reported higher levels of satisfaction in their relationship, and stayed together for longer. This shows us that laughter is an emotion that we can use with those with whom we are emotionally close, to make ourselves feel better.

This is critical to our enjoying a happy mood – but maybe even more important when our present circumstances are making us feel lonely and in need of some company.

Laughter requires precise timing.

In conversations, most people time their laughter to occur very precisely at the ends of sentences, but have you noticed that some just want to tell the punch line and ruin it?

Laughter is attractive.

Can you really laugh someone into bed? One study of personal dating adverts found that both men and women specified a sense of humour more frequently than intelligence, education, profession or sexual drive as a preferred quality they would ideally choose than others.

As one man's liberator is another man's terrorist, so is one person's description of their partner as having a great sense of humour to another person they are unfunny and very boring.

Eileen, Barbara, Deirdre, Carol, Pam, Uncle Len and my Mum made me laugh, although they have all died, the sound and the lovely feeling of their laughter is still very much alive in my mind and in my feelings of happiness.

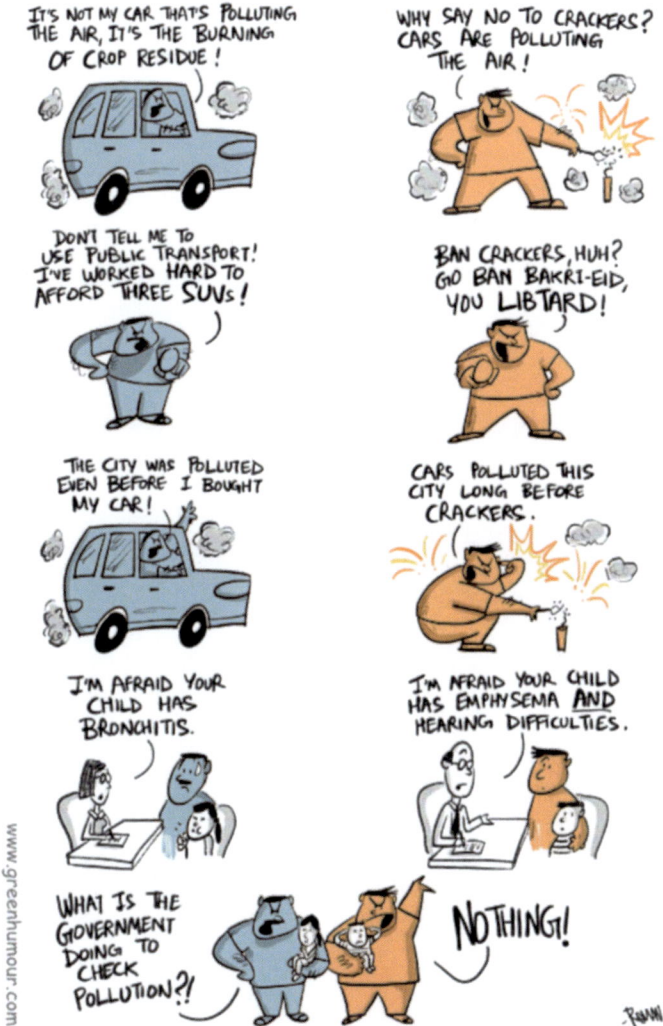

49. Love – What Is It and Can I Love in Different Ways?

I love you. Love is most likely to be used as a positive emotion with vastly differing degrees of intensity. We can say we love the sun, a particular food, the sea, a particular piece of music or a person. Many pledge their love to a partner or spouse until death do us part.

Four Greek words: *Eros*, *Storge*, *Philia*, and *Agape*. Romantic love, family love, brotherly love, and divine love.

Eros (Pronounced: AIR-ohs) is the Greek word for sensual or romantic love. The term originated from the mythological Greek goddess of love, sexual desire, physical attraction, and physical love.

Storge (Pronounced: STOR-jay) This Greek word describes family love, the affectionate bond that develops naturally between parents and children, and brothers and sisters.

Philia (Pronounced: FILL-ee-uh) is the type of intimate love the powerful emotional bond seen in deep friendships. Philia is the most general type of love, encompassing love for fellow humans, care, respect, and compassion for people in need. The concept of brotherly love that unites most of us.

Agape (Pronounced: Uh-GAH-pay) Agape love is perfect, unconditional, sacrificial, and pure.

Romantic love is made up of three elements:

1. **Attachment:** The need to be cared for and be with the other person. Physical contact and approval are also important components of attachment.
2. **Caring:** Valuing the other person's happiness and needs as much as your own.
3. **Intimacy:** Sharing private thoughts, feelings, and physical desires with the other person.

Self-love is also very important in the process of good mental health and psychotherapy.

No, it is not selfish to love yourself. It's about forgiving ourselves, warts and all.

"Love thy neighbour as thyself." No wonder that so many of us are so awful to our neighbours as few of us love ourselves! Do you?

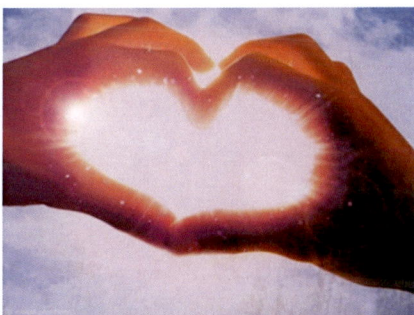

Who do you love, who loves you, who do you love that doesn't love you, who loves you but you don't love them?

Can you love more than one person, do you have different kinds of love and how do you behave when you feel someone doesn't love you?

What a lot of questions. What about answers, are there any?

Yes, start by loving yourself.

When you let go of who you are, you are able to find who you can be.

– Buddhist saying.

LOVE

Seeing we are in February in which Valentine's day presents us with the many opportunities we have to express our love outwardly with cards, (maybe some secretly) flowers and/or chocolates, let us look at love.

The opposite to love is fear. Yes, the opposite of love is not, as we many times, or almost always think, hatred, but the fear to love, and fear to love is the fear of being free. So it was of no surprise that many were fearful of the possibility of contacting any infection by being with other people, at the long agreed time of the pantomime.

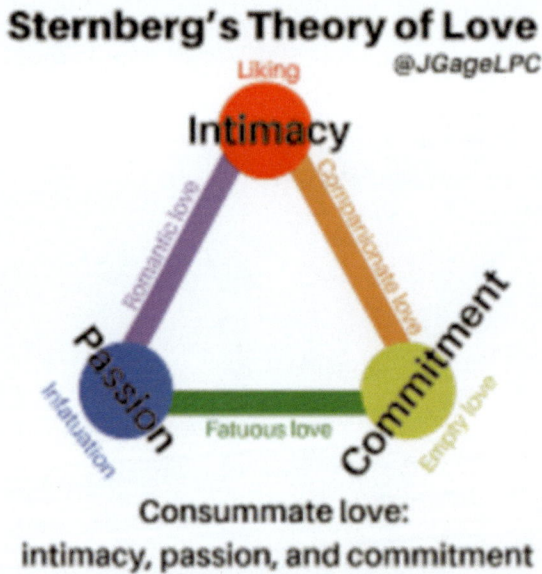

Sternberg's Theory of Love

@JGageLPC

Liking

Intimacy

Romantic love

Companionate love

Passion

Infatuation

Fatuous love

Commitment

Empty love

Consummate love:
intimacy, passion, and commitment

Now, let us now look at Sternberg's Theory of Love.

The love in the pantomime group is rife. However, according to this theory it is named empty love which to me sounds negative but if that is the given category for the state of commitment love, then it is true; because the commitment of what so many people have given to the rehearsals and to each other has been eye-opening. What could have become a no goer because of Covid-19 pandemic has in fact emerged to offer an even more committed group of children and adults producing, I hope, many fun performances.

Interesting isn't it that the postponement of it has made many of the cast even keener to be involved. Like you don't appreciate something until it is taken away.

Rather like taking for granted your electricity, water, boiler or garden plants, only then realizing how much we loved such things, if we lose them.

Passion is self-explanatory. We can be passionate about our values, our politics. our religion, our hobbies, our consumer durables but the passion of love, be it romantic love, infatuation or fatuous love I guess, without any evidence, is by far the preferred passion for almost everybody.

Intimacy is not just a physical state but a mental feeling of wellbeing. Remember, Intimacy is Game free. You don't have to plan what you are going to say; you don't have to avoid being truthful with the fear of it being used against you; you know you will not be judged but accepted. When relationships are game free you are intimate.

50. My Mind Makes Me Mentally Well

Do you believe that there is such a thing as psychosomatic illness?

You do? In which case is there such a thing then as psychosomatic wellness?

There certainly is. How many times have you talked yourself into not feeling well enough to go into work or college, as an excuse, when really you were fine but as the day progressed you did start to feel ill, thinking yourself unwell?

If you think you are well, you are well.

How? The starting point is to begin by loving our self.

No, that does not mean being selfish and inconsiderate of others.

It means forgiving ourselves of things that we might have done for which we feel ashamed or regret or what we might not have done that we wish that we had. We need to love ourselves warts and al.

Now let us think about **trust**.

When trust gets broken it virtually never gets back to what it was.

Well hardly ever, but maybe you have been able to trust again.

Who do you trust?

To be your husband, wife, partner, lover, or confidential friend?

To support you when life becomes scary or stressful?

To keep your confidence?

Many of us may have a fear of betrayal or loss because of our past experiences. Sadly, with the increase of divorcees, their children are likely to grow up with a resistance of full commitment to a partner and have a fear of trusting again and a fear of betrayal because subconsciously they do not want to be vulnerable and hurt again

When we feel negative emotions, we are less likely to trust others.

We may base our decisions about whom to trust on their attractiveness, how much they resemble our kin members, and their facial features.

People may have a 'preconscious friend-or-foe mental mechanism' that helps them to evaluate others during interactions (*partners* are usually trusted more than *opponents*).

Trust in strangers increases from childhood to early adulthood, and then remains more or less stable in adulthood.

Trustworthiness is an esteemed virtue among friends and employers alike and it comes with a host of perks. Those with more trust are less likely to lie, and appear more ethical, more attractive and even happier. Someone, who is deemed trustworthy appears to epitomise a set of positive characteristics including ability and benevolence, the will to do good.

A person with trust issues may harbour negative beliefs about trust and may find themselves thinking limiting thoughts, such as:

'I can never let my guard down again.'
'If I open up to this new lover I will only get hurt again.'
'Everyone is out to get me.'

These barriers are often a person's way of avoiding the rejection, pain or guilt that is associated with mistrust.

Without trust you cannot have love, so try trusting again.

If you always do what you've always done
You'll always get what you've always got –
So, try something different – trust.
Try changing what were painful emotions now into painful memories.

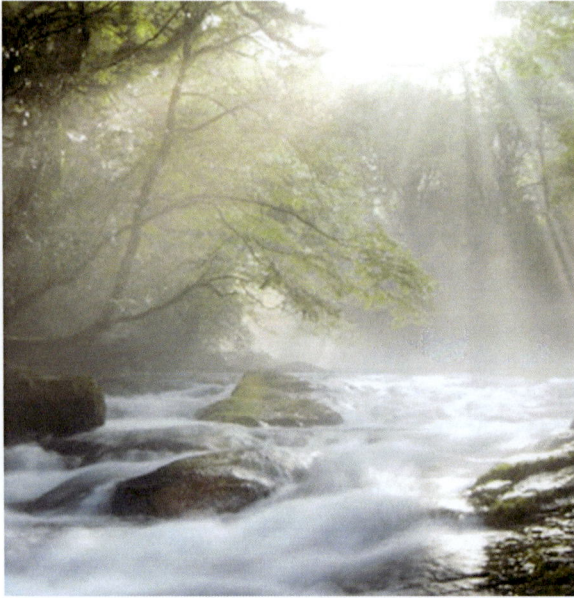

Changing Painful Emotions into Painful Memories

Almost all of us may have had to grieve for the loss of a loved one. We may experience a range of emotions. Guilt, loneliness, disbelief, abandonment, loss, fear, depression, anger, although that is often not expressed.

"How can I be angry, they didn't mean to die". Also relief, again not easily admitted but nevertheless is often felt when you have watched someone you dearly love suffering from a painful illness, for instance cancer.

In bereavement counselling there are several theories about the stages of bereavement. Firstly, **Denial**, you cannot believe that it has happened, especially when it is sudden. Then A**nger**. **Bargaining**, is another stage, *'if only' I had done this, or he or she hadn't done that.* Also, **Depression,** *without that person in my life, how will I cope?* Finally, A**cceptance** or adaption when we know and accept that the loved one is dead and will not return.

However, these are not chronological stages one to five. In fact, they need to be thought of as aspects of bereavement because we can feel depressed one day, then accepting and then angry on another day followed by denial or any other of the other various stages and experience other emotional states. There is no order of stages.

Many things, a song, a play, a book, a name, a place or someone's comment can trigger off a painful emotion.

The word closure, is so often used, which really is acceptance. Particularly relevant for families of missing persons. Then we can see beyond the death and start to remember their life as a whole.

In terms of 'getting better' research shows that when fighting a legal case for compensation or a decision, this can delay recovery. Hence having to wait, sometimes years, for legal decisions, like Hillsborough, Shoreham air disaster, creates such stress.

Also we may need to grieve for the loss of someone through separation, divorce, a miscarriage, illness, addiction, or mental health difficulties of a loved one. Or their physical health difficulties may have profoundly changed them because of an accident or injury.

Grieving is a process not a single act. Grieving takes as long as it takes and is not about achieving 'closure'. We have **continuing bonds** with those who have died and these bonds may be crucial in sustaining us through the pain of loss. Think of the continuing bonds you have with someone.

Grief is the price we pay for love. Without attachment there would be no sense of loss. Whatever your religious beliefs, or none, are about everlasting life, your time and experience spent with that person, the memory of their love and how they influenced you, will be everlasting.

It is important to give yourself permission to grieve, it is also important to give yourself permission to be happy.

Remember using the word **'died'**, not lost, passed on, left me or other terms that people constantly use for death, as this helps with the important stage of healing **accepting** that they have died.

We cannot change the painful experience but we can change it into a painful memory. We can celebrate the love we had then, bring it into the now and pass it on.

51. On Acceptance not Closure

So many times, we hear the media talk about 'now you have closure'. We don't want closure, we want acceptance. Because when someone that we love, dies we want to be able to recall our special memories, which can be triggered by so many incidental things; a comment, music, a book, TV, a play, hearing their name, recalling a part of their life. It is not until we reach an acceptance stage, in the grieving process that we can begin to celebrate our memories.

Such sadness around in the death of Pam Finch. Her humour, love and kindness were infectious. As she said to me in the last panto, 'I started as the back end of a cow and look at me now, I have progressed to going on stage in my underwear.'

We have just had Easter in an atmosphere of such suffering with so many deaths due to the Coronavirus epidemic, when so many thousands of people will be grieving. There would be no Christians if we had had closure on Good Friday, Christians would not want closure but the acceptance that Christ rose from the dead.

For many of us we are in lock down with time to think rather than being involved in our usual frantic activity. Our life is made up of time so waste your time and you waste your life. The psyche is very powerful and you can use it positively or negatively.

We have a feeling brain and a thinking brain; the feeling brain is greater that the thinking brain when we are feeling a lot of emotion the thinking brain can shut down. Do you believe that how you think affects how you feel? Yes? Then do you believe that how you feel affects how you think? Yes? Then do you believe that how you feel affects how you behave? Yes? So, thinking and feeling positively and being appreciative for what is being done for us, is likely to affect how we behave towards others and towards ourselves.

In these times of so much death in Ukraine whilst we need to give ourselves permission to grieve, we also need to give ourselves permission to be happy in the memory of our loved ones.

We do not want closure we want acceptance to celebrate the love, if we had it, not to continuing mourn the loss.

Whichever religion we follow, or whether we are an agnostic or an atheist, almost all of us can find comfort in the belief of the everlasting life of our memories.

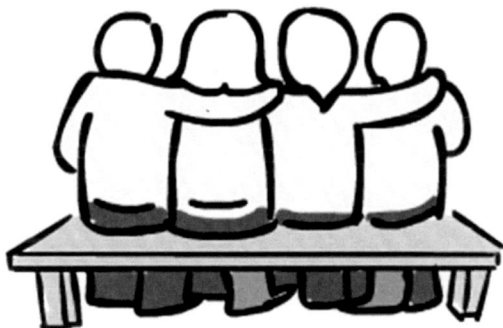

Friendship

Many people feel lonely after a celebratory time or when a holiday is over, do you?
What wonderful friendship you experienced over the festive celebrations or holiday?
New friends are fun you have a fresh sheet to start your thumbnail sketch of your life.
Here are a few thoughts about friendship from a diverse source of quotes.

"A friend listens to the music behind the words and doesn't join in with 'me, me, me' and never says 'I told you so'. He or she is always there for sharing **Love, Illness, Fear and Enjoyment**."

–Jeanie Civil

"Friendship is unnecessary, like philosophy, like art... It has no survival value; rather it is one of those things that give value to survival."

–C.S. Lewis

"Most of us don't need a psychiatric therapist as much as a friend to be silly with."

–Robert Brault

"Only your real friends will tell you when your face is dirty."

–Sicilian Proverb

"The antidote for fifty enemies is one friend."

–Aristotle

"A loyal friend laughs at your jokes when they're not so good, and sympathises with your problems when they're not so bad."

–Arnold H. Glasgow

"The friend is the man who knows all about you, and still likes you."

–Elbert Hubbard, The Notebook, 1927

"If a friend is in trouble, don't annoy him by asking if there is anything you can do. Think up something appropriate and do it."

–Edgar Watson Howe

"The most beautiful discovery true friends make is that they can grow separately without growing apart."

–Elisabeth Foley

"It is easier to forgive an enemy than to forgive a friend."

–William Blake

"If a man does not make new acquaintances as he advances through life, he will soon find himself alone. A man should keep his friendships in constant repair."

–Samuel Johnson

"Some people go to priests; others to poetry; I to my friends."

–Virginia Woolf